PARAMEDIC
CRASH COURSE®

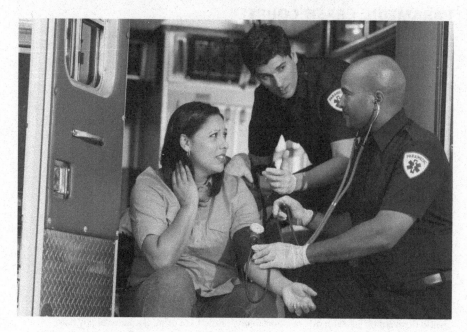

Chris Coughlin, NRP, Ph.D.

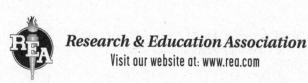

Research & Education Association
Visit our website at: www.rea.com

Research & Education Association
1325 Franklin Ave., Suite 250
Garden City, NY 11530
Email: info@rea.com

PARAMEDIC CRASH COURSE®

Published 2022
Copyright © 2019 by Research & Education Association.
All rights reserved. No part of this book may be reproduced
in any form without permission of the publisher.

Printed in the United States of America

Library of Congress Control Number 2018959978

ISBN-13: 978-0-7386-1246-1
ISBN-10: 0-7386-1246-4

TABLE of CONTENTS

PART I

PHARMACOLOGY

PART II

AIRWAY/ASSESSMENT/BLEEDING AND SHOCK

PART III

MEDICAL EMERGENCIES UNIT 1

MEDICAL EMERGENCIES UNIT 2

PART V — TRAUMA

PART VI — SPECIAL PATIENTS

PART VII — EMS OPERATIONS

ONLINE PRACTICE EXAM.... *available at www.rea.com/studycenter*

ABOUT OUR BOOK

REA's *Paramedic Crash Course* is designed for the last-minute studier or any prospective candidate who wants a quick refresher before taking the National Paramedic Certification Exam. Our *Crash Course* will show you how to study efficiently and strategically, so you can pass your exam.

Written by a veteran EMS Program Director and NREMT paramedic, REA's *Paramedic Crash Course* gives you a review specifically targeted to what you really need to know to ace the exam.

- Our **Introduction** discusses the requirements for becoming a Paramedic, exam information including the topics covered, as well as test-taking tips for succeeding on the exam.

- **Part I** reviews Pharmacology and metrics and drug calculations.

- **Parts II, III, IV, and V** cover patient assessment, resuscitation, trauma, and medical and environmental emergencies.

- **Part VI** explains special patient care, with special attention to pediatric and geriatric patients.

- **Part VII** reviews EMS operations, such as ambulance and air medical operations.

- The **Appendix** provides valuable tips to help you prepare for the psychomotor exam.

ABOUT OUR PRACTICE EXAM

Are you ready for the exam? Find out by taking REA's online practice exam available at *www.rea.com/studycenter*. This true-to-format practice test features automatic scoring and detailed explanations of all answers. It will help you identify your strengths and weaknesses so you'll be ready on exam day.

Good luck on your Paramedic certification exam!

A LETTER FROM OUR AUTHOR

This book is intended for current paramedic students and recent graduates who will be sitting for the national certification exam. Your primary paramedic text is probably 2,000+ pages and impossible to memorize. This *Paramedic Crash Course* is not meant to replace that resource. Nonetheless this *Crash Course* book is considerably more concise than your paramedic text (good news) and focuses on providing you with the must-know information needed to pass the certification exam. This book is based on a few presumptions:

1. You are completing, or have completed, a high-quality programmatically accredited paramedic education program.

2. You completed a human anatomy and physiology course either before or during your paramedic education program.

3. You are proficient at ECG interpretation.

4. You are knowledgeable about the current American Heart Association guidelines for Basic Life Support and Advanced Cardiac Life Support.

Listen carefully to any advice provided by your paramedic education program core instructors, program director, and medical director. These experts know you, your strengths and weaknesses, and your dominant learning style. Your program also has access to information regarding how its graduates have historically performed on the certification exam. Their NREMT pass rates are most likely available on their website, or upon request.

You should be able to review this book, memorize the material you agree is important and don't already know, and complete the included practice exam in 30 days or less. The good news is you don't need to be an academic all-star, or a brilliant test-taker, to get ready for the national certification exam (most of us who passed this exam are neither of those things). You just need a genuine desire to help others and a strong work ethic.

Study hard. Good luck. Be safe!

Chris Coughlin

NRP, Ph.D.

ABOUT OUR AUTHOR

Dr. Chris Coughlin is the Department Chair for Public Safety Sciences at Glendale Community College in Glendale, Arizona.

Dr. Coughlin has been a nationally certified paramedic since 1991 and was one of the first 850 nationally certified (FP-C) flight paramedics in the United States.

Dr. Coughlin earned his AAS in Advanced Emergency Medical Technology from Glendale Community College; his B.A. in Adult Education from Ottawa University; his M.Ed. in Educational Leadership from Northern Arizona University; and his Ph.D. in Education from Capella University.

Dr. Coughlin welcomes correspondence at *chris.coughlin@gccaz.edu*

AUTHOR DEDICATION AND ACKNOWLEDGMENTS

Dedicated to my children, Saren, Alissa, Hannah, and Nathan, who I am proud to watch as they pursue their own paths.

Special thanks to Diane Goldschmidt, REA Managing Editor, who championed this project and made it happen; Lead Reviewer Daniel Fitzpatrick, for his invaluable input; and all the Subject Matter Experts listed below who contributed significantly to this project.

Lead Reviewer

Daniel Fitzpatrick, Firefighter, NRP
EMS Training Division, Glendale Fire Department
Adjunct Faculty, Glendale Community College
Glendale, Arizona

Subject Matter Experts

Will Burner, BS, NRP
Captain, Paramedic, Terrorism Liaison Officer
Glendale Fire Department, Glendale, Arizona

George Cantini, MS, PA
Emergency Medicine Physician Assistant
Residential Faculty
Glendale Community College, Glendale, Arizona

David Cleveland, BS, NRP
Battalion Chief, El Mirage Fire Department, El Mirage, Arizona
Paramedic Program Coordinator,
Glendale Community College, Glendale, Arizona

Robert Dotterer, BSEd, M.Ed, NRP
Program Director, Paramedicine
Paradise Valley Community College, Phoenix, Arizona

Troy R. Lutrick, MS, NRP, CEM
Division Chief, Emergency Management, Homeland Security
City of Avondale Fire and Medical, Avondale, Arizona

Rainier Perez, BA NRP
Battalion Commander
Albuquerque Fire Department (retired)
Albuquerque, New Mexico

Todd Polansky, BA, NRP
Paramedic Program Director
Glendale Community College, Glendale, Arizona

Peter W. Vann, MD FACEP
Emergency Physician (retired)
Adjunct Faculty, Paramedic Program
Glendale Community College, Glendale, Arizona

Ian Winterstein, NRP
Firefighter, Paramedic
Glendale Fire Department, Glendale, Arizona

ABOUT REA

Founded in 1959, Research & Education Association (REA) is dedicated to publishing the finest and most effective educational materials—including study guides and test preps—for students of all ages.

Today, REA's wide-ranging catalog is a leading resource for students, teachers, and other professionals. Visit *www.rea.com* to see a complete listing of all our titles.

Introduction
Preparing for Success on the National Paramedic Certification Exam

Serving the public as a paramedic is an extremely demanding and rewarding career. Most states in the United States require that candidates pass the rigorous testing process of the National Registry of Emergency Medical Technicians (NREMT) to be eligible to work as a paramedic. Your future patients don't care what you scored on a test. They care about receiving competent and compassionate care for themselves and those they care about. Certification through the NREMT indicates to the public that you have demonstrated competency as a paramedic. This *Crash Course* gives you the essential information you need to prepare for the certification exam and your new career.

 REQUIREMENTS FOR BECOMING A PARAMEDIC

1. Be 18 years of age or older.

2. Hold a current NREMT certification or state license at the EMT level or higher.

3. Have successfully completed, within the past 2 years, a Paramedic program that has been accredited by the Commission on Accreditation of Allied Health Education Programs (CAAHEP), or a program that has a CAAHEP "Letter of Review." The Program Director of the course you take must verify your successful completion of the course through the NREMT website.

4. Have a current CPR-BLS for "Healthcare Provider" or equivalent credential.

5. Successfully complete the NREMT cognitive (knowledge) and psychomotor (skills) exams.

 THE EXAM

The National Paramedic Certification exam is a computer-adaptive test (CAT). This means that you take the test using a computer, and that an algorithm adjusts the exam to your maximum ability level in real time as you are taking the test. The exam delivers questions one at a time and the questions are not randomly chosen. Instead, the test tailors itself to your individual abilities. While you are taking the test, the software that drives the test is estimating your ability level. The ability estimate gets more and more precise as the exam progresses. The exam ends when there is a 95% certainty that your demonstrated competency is above or below the passing standard. It is unlikely any two candidates will take the same exact test; however, all candidates will take a test that meets the same test plan.

The exam complies with the Americans with Disabilities Act (ADA) with regard to requests for examination accommodations consistent with its mission and public protection.

III. TOPICS COVERED ON THE EXAM

Your exam will most likely have at least 80 and no more than 150 questions. You will have 2 hours and 30 minutes to complete the test. Less than 1% of candidates are unable to finish the exam in the time allowed. Take the time to read every question carefully. The exam will include traditional multiple-choice style questions and may have so-called technology-enhanced items, or TEIs. Examples of TEIs include:

- Multiple-response items (direct you to select more than one correct answer option)
- Graphic images
- Highlighting or matching
- Ordered response
- Video-enhanced questions

The NREMT identifies several advantages to including these types of questions. TEIs can make the test more authentic and engaging, better simulate working in the field, and better test critical-thinking skills. For more information about TEIs on the national certification exam, visit *http://www.nremt.org*.

The exam will broadly cover the content of the current National EMS Education Standards (NEMSES) and the current American Heart Association *Guidelines for Cardiopulmonary Resuscitation and Emergency Cardiovascular Care*. Correct answers are based on national standards, not local or state protocols. The exam emphasizes questions about what a Paramedic should do in the field, so you should expect a lot of scenario-based questions.

Topics will include airway, respiration and ventilation, cardiology and resuscitation, trauma, medical emergencies, obstetrics, gynecology, and EMS operations. The table below shows the percentages for the topics found on the exam.

NREMT Test Plan for Paramedic Candidates

Content Area	Percent of Exam
Airway, Respiration & Ventilation	18%–22%
Cardiology & Resuscitation	22%–26%
Trauma	13%–17%
Medical; Obstetrics & Gynecology	25%–29%
EMS Operations	10%–14%

Source: https://www.nremt.org/rwd/public/document/cognitive-exam

For all but EMS operations, 85% of the questions relate to adult patients and 15% relate to pediatric patients. Although not separate categories, topics such as patient assessment, anatomy and physiology, pediatric emergencies, and safety will be emphasized throughout the test.

IV. SCORING

Typically, you can retrieve your score from your NREMT account within 2 business days after you complete the exam. If you fail the exam, the NREMT will provide some detailed information about your performance on each of the exam categories. Candidates must wait at least 15 days before taking the test again.

V. STANDARDS

Like the certification exam, the information in this publication is based on the current National EMS Education Standards (NEMSES) and the current American Heart Association *Guidelines for Cardiopulmonary Resuscitation and Emergency Cardiovascular Care (CPR & ECC Guidelines).*

This *Crash Course* will help you become familiar with these standards before taking the certification exam; however, you should not rely on any one resource to prepare for the exam.

For more information about the current NEMSES, visit *https://www.ems.gov/education.html.*

For more information about the current American Heart Association Guidelines, visit *https://eccguidelines.heart.org.*

VI. GENERAL TEST-TAKING TIPS AND STRATEGIES

- Try to take your NREMT exam soon after finishing your paramedic course. Strive to take the test within 30 days of completing your program. The longer you wait to take the exam, the less likely you are to pass.

- Study regularly over an extended period before the test. Don't cram. Your preparation should end (not begin) the day before the test.

- Avoid caffeine, energy drinks, excess sugar, etc. These will not improve your performance or steady your nerves.

- Know exactly where the test center is and plan to arrive early. Remember, you must have an appointment to take the test. Bring two forms of photo ID.

- Dress comfortably so you are not distracted by being too hot or too cold while taking the test. And don't show up for the test hungry, tired, or otherwise unfocused.

VII. DURING THE TEST

- You *cannot* skip a question or come back to it later. You must answer each question before the next one will be provided.

- Read the whole question thoroughly at least a couple of times and formulate the answer in your head before you look at the answer choices. If you see a similar answer choice, that's probably the correct response.

- There are four answer choices. Two of them can often be eliminated after reading the question thoroughly. There is only one "best" answer.

- When you get stuck, look for key words in the question and reread the answer choices. When in doubt, lean toward the more aggressive treatment. For example, if you are not sure whether you should ventilate the patient or just administer oxygen, choose to ventilate.

- Do not complicate scenario-based questions. Do not bring elements into the questions that are not there.

- Relax! Remember, everyone is going to feel like the test is extremely challenging. Everyone is going to miss questions. This does NOT mean you are failing.

PART I

PHARMACOLOGY

Medication Administration/ Drug Calculations

I. TERMS TO KNOW

A. Bioavailability—the amount of a drug that enters central circulation and is able to cause an effect

B. Bolus—administration of medication in single dose (as opposed to an infusion)

C. Concentration—for calculation purposes, this is the total amount of medication available as packaged, e.g., total amount of drug (mcg, mg, g) in the syringe, ampule, etc.

D. Dose—the drug amount intended for administration

E. Enteral—delivery of medication through the GI tract (oral, sublingual, rectal)

F. Half-life—period of time required for concentration of drug in the body to be reduced by one-half

G. LD50—Lethal dose (LD50) is the amount of an ingested substance (in mg/kg) that kills 50% of a test sample

H. Parenteral—delivery of medication outside of the GI tract, e.g., IV, IO, IM, SQ, intranasal

I. Pharmacokinetics—movement of a drug through the body, includes absorption, bioavailability, distribution, metabolism, and excretion

J. Pharmacodynamics—the mechanism of action of a medication

K. Therapeutic index—the range between minimum effective dose of a medication and the maximum safe dose. The narrower the therapeutic index, the more risk associated with the medication.

L. Volume—for calculation purposes, this is the total amount of fluid available as packaged, e.g., total amount of fluid (mL) in the syringe, ampule, etc.

II. MEDICATION LEGISLATION

1. Pure Food and Drug Act (1906)—Prevents the manufacture, sale, or transportation of misbranded or poisonous medications.

2. Harrison Narcotic Act (1914)—Regulates production, importation, and distribution of opiates.

3. Federal Food, Drug, and Cosmetic Act (1938)—Gives the U.S. Food and Drug Administration authority to oversee the safety of food, drugs, and cosmetics.

4. Controlled Substances Act (1970)—Categorizes controlled substances based on their potential for abuse and potential medical benefits.

5. Schedules

   i. Schedule I

      ➤ high potential for abuse. No accepted medical use.

      ➤ Examples: heroin, LSD, ecstasy, peyote

   ii. Schedule II

      ➤ narcotics and stimulants with high potential for abuse and severe dependence

      ➤ Examples: methadone, morphine, codeine, amphetamine, methamphetamine

   iii. Schedule III

      ➤ less potential for abuse, can still cause low physical or high psychological dependence

      ➤ Examples: Vicodin, acetaminophen with codeine, ketamine, anabolic steroids

   iv. Schedule IV

      ➤ low potential for abuse

      ➤ Examples: Xanax, Soma, Valium, Ativan, Versed, Ambien

  v.   Schedule V

  ➤ contains limited quantities of narcotics, such as cough syrups with codeine

III. AVOIDING MEDICATION ERRORS

A. The Six Rights of Drug Administration

1. Right patient

2. Right drug

3. Right time

4. Right route

5. Right amount

6. Right documentation

B. Keep similarly packaged drugs separated in drug box, such as ampules of epinephrine and morphine.

C. Always confirm medication and dose with fellow EMS provider.

D. If you pull it or draw it up, you administer it.

E. Confirm dosage with appropriate reference sources (AHA guidelines, state standards, agency protocols, etc.).

IV. COMMON PREHOSPITAL ROUTES OF MEDICATION ADMINISTRATION

A. Enteral (through the GI tract)

1. Oral

2. Rectal

B. Parenteral (outside of the GI tract)

1. Subcutaneous

2. Intramuscular

3. Intravenous

4. Intraosseous

5. Sublingual

6. Nasal

7. Inhaled

V. DRUG CALCULATIONS

A. Metrics review

1. Liter (measure of volume)

    i. 1,000 milliliters (mL) = 1 Liter

        Note: 1 mL = 1 cubic centimeter (cc)

2. Gram (measure of weight)

    i.   1,000 micrograms (mcg) = 1 milligram (mg)

    ii. 1,000 mg = 1 gram

    iii. 1,000 grams = 1 kilogram (kg)

    iv. 1 kg = 2.2 pounds (lbs)

B. Bolus calculations

1. (volume of fluid in mL × desired dose in mg) ÷ concentration (the total amount of drug as packaged) = mL to administer

    i.   Above formula can also be expressed as: $\dfrac{V \times D}{C} = mL$

    ii. **Example:** You are ordered to administer 0.5 mg of atropine using a 1 mg/10 mL syringe.

         Volume = 10 mL

         Dose = 0.5 mg

         Concentration = 1 mg

         $\dfrac{10 \times 0.5}{1} = 5$ mL

    iii. **Example:** You are ordered to administer 1 mg per kg of lidocaine to a 50 kg patient using a 100 mg/5 mL syringe.

         Volume = 5 mL

         Dose = 50 mg (50 kg × 1)

Concentration = 100 mg

$$\frac{5 \times 50}{100} = 2.5 \text{ mL}$$

iv. **Example:** You are ordered to administer 2 mg of diazepam using a 10 mg/2 mL syringe.

Volume = 2 mL

Dose = 2 mg

Concentration = 10 mg

$$\frac{2 \times 2}{10} = 0.4 \text{ mL}$$

C. IV infusions

1. IV tubing drop factors (drops per mL)

   i. Macrodrip tubing = typically 10 drops per mL (may also be 15 or 20)

   ii. Microdrip (pediatric) tubing = 60 drops per mL

2. IV infusion calculations (no medications added)

   i. $\dfrac{\text{Ordered volume (mL)} \times \text{IV tubing drop factor}}{\text{Minutes}}$ = drops per minute

   ii. **Example:** 150 mL per hour with macrodrip tubing

   Ordered vol: = 150

   Drop factor = 10

   Minutes = 60

   $$\frac{150 \times 10}{60} = 25 \text{ drops per min}$$

   iii. **Example:** 65 mL per hour with microdrip tubing

   Ordered vol: = 65

   Drop factor = 60

   Minutes = 60

   $$\frac{65 \times 60}{60} = 65 \text{ drops per min}$$

D. IV Medication Infusions (medication added to IV bag)

1.
$$\frac{\text{Volume of IV bag} \times \text{Dose of med ordered} \times \text{Tubing drop factor}}{\text{Concentration (total amt of drug in IV bag)} \times \text{Minutes}} = \text{drops per min}$$

2. **Example:** Administer 2 mg per minute of lidocaine with microdrip tubing using 1 gram (1,000 mg) of lido in 250 mL IV.

Volume = 250 mL

Dose = 2

Tubing = 60

Concentration = 1,000 (dose is in mg, so concentration must also be in mg)

Minutes = 1

$$\frac{250 \times 2 \times 60}{1,000 \times 1} = 30 \text{ drops per min}$$

3. **Example:** Administer 5 mcg per kg per minute of dopamine using microdrip tubing with 400 mg of dopamine in 250 mL IV. Patient weight is 90 kg.

Volume = 250

Dose = 450 (90 kg x 5)

Tubing = 60

Concentration = 400,000 (Dose and concentration must both be in mg or mcg. Can't have one in mg and the other in mcg.)

Minutes = 1

$$\frac{250 \times 450 \times 60}{400,000 \times 1} = 17 \text{ drops per min}$$

Calculations	
How many mcg (μg) per mg?	1,000 mcg (μg) per mg
How many mg per gram?	1,000 mg per gram
How many pounds per kg?	2.2 lbs per kg
How many mL per liter?	1,000 mL per liter
What is the drop factor for: ➤ Blood tubing ➤ Macro (Adult) tubing ➤ Pediatric tubing	**Blood** (a "macro" tubing) = 10 drops per mL **Macro (not blood)** AKA "regular" or "adult" tubing = Variable drip rate (10, 15, 20 drops per mL) **Pediatric** "micro" tubing = 60 drops per mL
What is the abbreviation for drop and drops?	Drop = gtt Drops = gtts
What is the formula for calculating a bolus medication?	$$\frac{\text{Volume} \times \text{Dose}}{\text{Concentration}} = \text{mL needed}$$ **Ex:** give 3 mg of Valium — **Volume** = 2 mL **Packaging:** 10 mg in 2 mL — **Dose** = 3 mg — **Concentration** = 10 mg $(2 \times 3) \div 10 = \textbf{0.6 mL}$
What is the formula for calculating a plain IV infusion rate?	$$\frac{\text{Ordered Volume} \times \text{Drop Factor}}{\text{Minutes}} = \text{drops per minute}$$ **Ex:** 100 mL per hour with 10 drop tubing $(100 \times 10) \div 60 = \textbf{17 drops per min}$

What is the formula for calculating an IV medication infusion?	$$\frac{\text{Volume} \times \text{Dose} \times \text{Drop Factor}}{\text{Concentration} \times \text{Minutes}} =$$ **drops per minute**

Ex: give 5 mcg/kg/min of dopamine (90 kg patient) **Pkg:** 400 mg in 250 mL	**Volume** = 250 mL **Dose** = 450 mcg (5 × 90) **Tubing** = 60 (peds) **Concentration** = 400 mg **Minutes** = 1

Note: The dose and concentration must match (both mg or both mcg). You can convert dose from 450 mg to .450 mcg or convert concentration from 400 mg to 400,000 mcg

$$(250 \times .450 \times 60) \div (400 \times 1) =$$
17 drops per min

Practice: plain IV infusions

Use 60 gtts peds tubing for 1–5:	Use 10 gtts blood tubing for 6–10:	Use 15 gtts adult tubing for 11–15:				
1) 110 mL/hr	6) 110 mL/hr	11) 110 mL/hr	1) 110 gtts/min	6) 18 gtts/min	11) 28 gtts/min
2) 65 mL/hr	7) 65 mL/hr	12) 65 mL/hr	2) 65 gtts/min	7) 11 gtts/min	12) 16 gtts/min
3) 80 mL/hr	8) 80 mL/hr	13) 80 mL/hr	3) 80 gtts/min	8) 13 gtts/min	13) 20 gtts/min
4) 200 mL/hr	9) 200 mL/hr	14) 200 mL/hr	4) 200 gtts/min	9) 33 gtts/min	14) 50 gtts/min
5) 150 mL/hr	10) 150 mL/hr	15) 150 mL/hr	5) 150 gtts/min	10) 25 gtts/min	15) 38 gtts/min

What are the shortcuts for plain IV flow rate calculations?	As long as the order is over an hour, divide it by:

➤ 6 for blood tubing

➤ 4 for adult (15 gtts) tubing

➤ 1 for peds tubing

100 mL per hr (blood tubing) = 100 ÷ 6 = **17 drops/min**

100 mL per hr (adult tubing) = 100 ÷ 4 = **25 drops/min**

100 mL per hr (peds tubing) = 100 ÷ 1 = **100 drops/min**

Practice: bolus calculations

1) atropine 0.5 mg use prefilled syringe	6) atropine 1.2 mg use multi-dose vial	11) Lasix 80 mg
2) Cordarone 300 mg	7) morphine 2 mg	12) lidocaine 60 mg
3) verapamil 2.5 mg	8) Benadryl 25 mg	13) Valium 2 mg
4) etomidate 24 mg	9) 10 grams of D$_{50}$	14) calcium 300 mg
5) sodium bicarb 20 mEq	10) Succinyl-choline 120 mg	15) 1.4 mg epi use 1:1,000 concen-tration

1) 5 mL	6) 3 mL	11) 8 mL
2) 6 mL	7) 0.2 mL	12) 3 mL
3) 1 mL	8) 0.5 mL	13) 0.4 mL
4) 12 mL	9) 20 mL	14) 3 mL
5) 20 mL	10) 6 mL	15) 1.4 mL

Practice: IV medication infusions

Lido Infusions: Use 1g/ 250 mL mix	Epi Infusions: Use 1 mg/ 250 mL mix	Dopamine Infusions: Use 400 mg/ 250 mL mix
1) Lido at 2 mg/min	4) Epi at 4 mcg/min	7) Dopamine 5 mcg/kg/min (90 kg)
2) Lido at 3 mg/min	5) Epi at 6 mcg/min	8) Dopamine 7 mcg/kg/min (90 kg)
3) Lido at 4 mg/min	6) Epi at 8 mcg/min	9) Dopamine 10 mcg/kg/min (90 kg)

1) 30 gtts/min	4) 60 gtts/min	7) 17 gtts/min
2) 45 gtts/min	5) 90 gtts/min	8) 24 gtts/min
3) 60 gtts/min	6) 120 gtts/min	9) 34 gtts/min

Note: use pediatric tubing for all

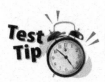

Test Tip

Good News! You will have access to an on-screen digital calculator during the test.

Drug Profiles

I. TERMS TO KNOW

A. Adrenergic—related to the sympathetic nervous system (think "adrenaline")

B. Adverse effect—unintended effect of a medication administration

C. Agonist—medication that stimulates a specific response

D. Analgesic—medication that reduces pain

E. Antagonist—medication that inhibits a specific action

F. Bolus—single dose of medication, given all at once

G. Cholinergic—related to the parasympathetic nervous system (think acetylcholine)

H. Contraindication—circumstance when a medication should not be used

I. Cumulative effect—repeated administration of a medication that produces effects that are more pronounced than the first dose

J. Drug class—categorization of medications with similarities or uses

K. Extra pyramidal—tremors, slurred speech, restlessness, muscle twitching, anxiety side effects

L. Habituation—diminishing of a physiological or emotional response to a frequently repeated stimulus, e.g., cigarettes

M. Hypersensitivity—undesirable reactions produced by the normal immune system, including allergies and autoimmunity

N. Hypertonic solution—solution that has a greater concentration of solutes on the outside of a cell when compared with the inside of a cell, causing fluid to move out of the cell

O. Hypotonic solution—solution that has a lesser concentration of solutes on the outside of a cell when compared with the inside of a cell, causing fluid to move into the cell

P. Indication—circumstance when a medication should be considered

Q. Isotonic solution—sodium concentration same as intracellular fluid

R. Mechanism of action—pharmacological effects of a medication

S. Potentiation—interaction between two or more medications causing a response greater than the sum of each individual medication

T. Refractory—resistant to treatment

U. Side effect—any unwanted effect of medication administration

V. Therapeutic action—desirable effects of medication administration

W. Tolerance—reduced response to a medication due to repeated use

X. Untoward effect—adverse or harmful side effects of medication administration

 II. SOURCES FOR INFORMATION

A. United States Pharmacopeia (USP)

B. National Formulary (NF)

C. Physicians' Desk Reference (PDR)

D. Drug package inserts

E. State EMS authority

III. DRUG CATEGORIES AND COMMON MEDICATIONS

A. Altered LOC/OD
   1. Activated charcoal
   2. Dextrose
   3. Glucagon
   4. Nalmefene
   5. Naloxone
   6. Thiamine

B. Analgesics
   1. Fentanyl
   2. Morphine
   3. Nitrous oxide

C. Antidysrhythmics/Antiarrhythmics
   1. Adenosine
   2. Amiodarone
   3. Atropine
   4. Cardizem
   5. Lidocaine
   6. Verapamil

D. Cardiac
   1. Aspirin
   2. Bumetanide
   3. Dopamine

4. Epinephrine

5. Furosemide

6. Nitroglycerine

E. Electrolytes/misc

   1. Calcium

   2. Magnesium sulfate

   3. Ondansetron

   4. Oxygen

   5. Oxytocin

   6. Phenylephrine

   7. Promethazine

   8. Sodium bicarbonate

F. Respiratory

   1. Albuterol

   2. Atrovent

   3. Decadron

   4. Diphenhydramine

   5. Methylprednisolone

G. Sedation/seizure/paralytic

   1. Diazepam

   2. Etomidate

   3. Ketamine

   4. Lorazepam

   5. Midazolam

   6. Succinylcholine

IV. DRUG PROFILE INFORMATION

A. Drug name

B. Drug class/mechanism of action

C. Indications

D. Contraindications

E. Adverse effects

F. Dose

> *Note:* Drug dosages can vary widely by region.

V. RECEPTOR SITES

A. Alpha 1 — medications that stimulate alpha 1 receptor sites cause vasoconstriction.

B. Beta 1 — medications that stimulate beta 1 receptor sites cause increased heart rate (chronotrope), increased cardiac force of contraction (inotrope), and increased myocardial conduction (dromotrope).

C. Beta 2 — medications that stimulate beta 2 receptors cause bronchodilation.

D. Opioid — medications that stimulate opioid receptor sites cause CNS depression, analgesia.

VI. COMMON PARAMEDIC MEDICATIONS

Note: Pharmacology protocols can vary widely based on agency, region, medical direction, and state protocols, etc. The information below is meant to provide a sample of the drug profile information paramedic candidates are typically expected to know. All of the following medications are included in the NEMSES Paramedic Instructional Guidelines and should be considered fair game on the national certification exam. *Always* follow local guidelines regarding administration of medications.

A. Common medications include

1. Activated charcoal

2. Adenosine

3. Albuterol

4. Amiodarone

5. Aspirin

6. Atropine

7. Dextrose

8. Diazepam

9. Diltiazem

10. Diphenhydramine

11. Dopamine

12. Epinephrine

13. Fentanyl

14. Glucagon

15. Ipratropium bromide

16. Lidocaine

17. Lorazepam

18. Magnesium sulfate

19. Midazolam

20. Morphine

21. Naloxone

22. Nitroglycerine

23. Nitrous oxide

24. Oxygen

25. Oxytocin

26. Promethazine

27. Thiamine

ACTIVATED CHARCOAL

Name(s): Charcoal, Actidose

Class: Adsorbent

MOA: Reduces systemic absorption of toxins from GI tract

Packaging: 15, 25, 50 gram bottle

Indications: Recently ingested toxins

Contraindications

— Ingestion of caustics or hydrocarbons

— Decreased LOC

— Unstable airway

Adverse Reactions

— N&V

— Black stool

Dose

— Adults: 1–2 grams per kg (usual dose 30–60 grams)

— Peds: 0.5–1 gram per kg

— Note: use caution with activated charcoal that contains Sorbitol

ADENOSINE

Name(s): Adenocard

Class: Antidysrhythmic, endogenous nucleoside

MOA: Slows conduction through AV node, interrupts re-entry pathways, slows sinus rate

Packaging: 6 mg/2 mL vial or prefilled syringe

Indications

— SVT (not A-flutter or A-fib)

— Wide complex tachycardia of unknown origin unresponsive to amiodarone or lidocaine

Contraindications

— Sick sinus syndrome

— 2nd or 3rd degree AV blocks

— A-fib and A-flutter

— Note: caution in patients with asthma, those on Theophylline, Persantine, Tegretol, and cardiac transplant patients

Adverse Reactions

— CV: transient asystole, bradycardia, PVCs, palpitations, chest pain, hypotension

— Resp: dyspnea, hyperventilation, tightness in throat, bronchospasm

— CNS: dizzy, lightheaded, headache, paresthesias, blurred vision

— GI: nausea, metallic taste

Adult Dose

— Initial: 6 mg rapid IVP, immed 20 mL flush. AC vein preferred. Use port closest to patient, elevate arm during admin. Continuous ECG monitoring required

— Repeat: may repeat at 12 mg × two in 1–2 minutes if needed

Special Considerations

— Short half-life (10 seconds)

— Administer rapidly followed by immediate 20 mL flush

— Reoccurrence of tachydysrhythmia is common

ALBUTEROL

Name(s): Proventil, Ventolin

Class: Sympathomimetic, bronchodilator

MOA: Bronchodilation, decreases airway resistance

Packaging: 2.5 mg/3 mL unit dose (sulfite free)

Indications: Bronchospasm

Contraindications

— Known allergy

— Use caution in combination with other sympathomimetics due to potentiating effects

Adverse Reactions

— CV: dysrhythmias, tachycardia

— CNS: tremors, nervousness, restlessness

Adult Dose

— 2.5 mg in 3 mL unit dose via SVN or in-line with BVM

— May repeat per medical direction

— May be combined with ipratropium

AMIODARONE

Name(s): Cordarone, Pacerone

Class: Antidysrhythmic

MOA: Negative chronotrope, dilates coronary arteries

Packaging: 150 mg/3 mL ampules (50 mg/mL)

Indications

— VF/pulseless VT unresponsive to defib & epinephrine

— Wide complex tachycardia of unknown origin

— Stable VT

— Polymorphic V-tach

Contraindications

— Known allergy

— Bradycardia

— 2nd, 3rd degree block

— Cardiogenic shock

— Hypotension

— Pulmonary edema, CHF

Adverse Reactions

— CV: bradycardia, hypotension, asystole, heart block, CHF, Polymorphic V-tach associated with a prolonged QT interval

— GI: N&V

— Other: fever, headache, dizziness, flushing, salivation, photophobia

Adult Dose: cardiac arrest

— 300 mg IV/IO first dose

— Repeat 150 mg IV/IO in 3–5 min if no response

Adult Dose: tachydysrhythmias v-tach, wide complex tach, a-flutter, a-fib, SVT:

— 150 mg in 50 mL D_5W infused over 10 min.

Adult Dose: maintenance infusion

— 1 mg per minute IV infusion

— Ex: add 150 mg to 50 mL D_5W. Run at 20 gtts/min. with peds tubing **OR**

— Ex: add 50 mg to 50 mL D_5W. Run at 60 gtts/min with peds tubing

ACETYLSALICYLIC ACID

Name(s): Aspirin, Bufferin, ASA

Class: Analgesic, anti-pyretic, anti-inflammatory

MOA: Decreased platelet aggregation

Packaging: 81 & 325 mg tablets

Indications

— Suspected MI (chest pain, ECG changes)

— Unstable angina

— Pain, discomfort, or fever in adult patient only

Contraindications

— Known allergy

— Bleeding ulcer, hemorrhage, hemophilia

— Allergy to salicylates or other NSAIDs

— Children and adolescents

Adverse Reactions

— Use caution in patients with history of asthma

— Side effects rare in adults with single dose

Adult Dose

— Cardiac: 160–325 mg (2–4 pediatric chewable)

— Note: ASA has been linked to Reye's Syndrome in pediatric patients

ATROPINE

Name(s): Atropine

Class: Anticholinergic, parasympathetic blocker

MOA: Increased HR, decreased mucus production, bronchodilation

Packaging:

— 1 mg/10 mL prefilled syringe (0.1 mg/mL)

— 8 mg/20 mL multi-dose vial (0.4 mg per/mL)

Indications

— Symptomatic bradycardia

— Organophosphate poisoning

— Refractory bronchospasm

Contraindications

— Known allergy

— Acute angle closure glaucoma (rare condition, and a relative contraindication)

Adverse Reactions

— Tachydysrhythmias

— Ventricular irritability

— Angina

— Dry mouth

Adult Dose: symptomatic bradycardia

— 0.5 mg rapid IVP

— Can repeat as needed to a max dose of 3 mg

Adult Dose: organophosphate poisoning

— 2–5 mg IV, repeat every 5 min as needed (no max dose)

— 8 mg/20 mL multidose vial:

• 1 mL = 0.4 mg

• 2.5 mL = 1 mg

Peds Dose: bradycardia

— You MUST correct hypoxia first!

— Atropine is 3rd line for pediatrics (O_2 and epi first!)

— 0.02 mg/kg (min. 0.1 mg) IVP

Max single dose:
— Child: 0.5 mg
— Adolescent: 1 mg

Special Considerations
— Administering too small doses or administering too slowly may cause paradoxical bradycardia
— Not a cardiac arrest drug
— Use multi-dose vial for organophosphate, nerve agent
— Likely ineffective with 2nd degree type 2 or 3rd degree heart block

DEXTROSE

Name(s):
— D10 (10% solution) and
— D50 (50% solution)

Class: Carbohydrate, hyperglycemic

MOA: Increases blood glucose levels, short-term osmotic diuresis

Packaging
— D10: 1 gram per 10 mL
  • Ex: 25 grams/250 mL
— D50: 1 gram per 2 mL
  • Ex: 25 grams/50 mL prefilled syringe

Indications
— Known hypoglycemia
— Altered LOC or seizures of unknown etiology
— Hyperkalemia (in combination with sodium bicarbonate and calcium chloride)

Contraindications: Head injury
— Note: Do NOT withhold dextrose from stroke or TBI patients with known hypoglycemia.

Adverse Reactions
— Cerebral edema
— Increased ICP
— Tissue necrosis (if IV infiltrates)

Adult Dose: 12.5–50 grams IV

— Note: Many jurisdictions now recommend D10 instead of D50 for all patients due to risk of hyperglycemia, cerebral edema, and tissue necrosis.

Peds Dose

— 0.5–1 gram per kg of D10 solution over 20 min.

— To make/admin D10:

• Remove 50 mL from 250 mL IV bag and add 50 mL of D50

• Administer 5–10 mL per kg of D10

DIAZEPAM

Name(s): Valium

Class: Benzodiazepine

MOA: CNS depressant, anti-convulsant, sedation

Packaging: 10 mg/2 mL prefilled syringe (5mg per mL)

Indications

— Grand mal (generalized) seizures

— Transient sedation for medical procedures

— Delirium tremens

— Status epilepticus

Contraindications

— Known allergy

— Angle closure glaucoma (relative)

Adverse Reactions

— CV: bradycardia, hypotension

— Resp: resp. depression

— CNS: confusion, coma

— Other: burning at injection site, tissue necrosis from infiltration

Adult Dose

— IV: 2 mg increments slow IVP (do not exceed 2 mg per min)

— Note: for 10 mg/2 mL packaging: quickly calculate mL by doubling dose and moving decimal once left. Ex:

• 2 mg = 0.4 mL

• 6 mg = 1.2 mL

Peds Dose

— IV: 0.2–0.3 mg/kg over at least 3 min or until seizure subsides.

— Rectal (<6 years): 0.3–0.5 mg/kg rectally (slow)

DILTIAZEM

Name(s): Cardizem

Class: Calcium channel blocker

MOA: Negative inotrope, slows SA and AV conduction

Packaging: 5 mg per mL vials

Indications

— A-fib & A-flutter with rapid ventricular rate

— SVT refractory to adenosine

Contraindications

— Known allergy

— Hypotension

— MI or cardiogenic shock

— V-tach

— 2nd, 3rd degree AV block

— WPW and Sick Sinus Syndrome

— Beta blockers

Adverse Reactions

— CV: hypotension, bradycardia, heart block, chest pain, asystole

— GI: N&V

— CNS: headache, fatigue, drowsiness

Adult Dose

— Initial dose: 0.25 mg/kg (usually 20 mg) slow IVP over 2 min.

— If no response: repeat in 15 min. 0.35 mg/kg (usually 25 mg)

— Consider reduced dose for elderly patients

— Note: consider pretreatment with calcium chloride to reduce possible hypotension

DIPHENHYDRAMINE

Name(s): Benadryl

Class: Antihistamine, anticholinergic

MOA

- — Blocks histamine receptors
- — Reduced capillary permeability
- — Reduced vasodilation and bronchospasm
- — Anti-emetic

Packaging: 50 mg/1 mL vial

Indications

- — Anaphylaxis (after epi)
- — Extrapyramidal symptoms
- — N&V (consider ondansetron)

Contraindications

- — Known allergy
- — Angle closure glaucoma (relative)
- — Asthma (relative)
- — Nursing mothers

Adverse Reactions

- — CV: hypotension, palpitations, dysrhythmias
- — Resp: anaphylaxis, thickening bronchial secretions, wheezing
- — CNS: sedation, seizures
- — Children: paradoxical CNS excitation

Adult Dose: 25–50 mg slow IV or deep IM

DOPAMINE

Name(s): Intropin

Class: sympathomimetic

MOA

- — 1–2 mcg/kg/min: cerebral & renal vasodilation, increased urine output
- — 2–10 mcg/kg/min: increased cardiac output & BP
- — 10–20 mcg/kg/min: alpha effects, peripheral vasoconstriction, increase PVR & preload

Packaging

- — 400 mg/5 mL vial (must be added to 250 mL IV fluid) OR
- — 400 mg/250 mL premix bag

Indications

— Symptomatic bradycardia (not first line)

— Hemodynamically significant hypotension without hypovolemia (after fluid therapy)

Contraindications

— Hypovolemic shock

Adverse Reactions

— CV: dysrhythmias, hypotension (low dose), hypertension

— GI/GU: N&V, renal shutdown at higher doses

— Other: significant tissue necrosis from infiltration

Adult Dose

— Mix: 400 mg in 250 mL (1,600 mcg/mL)

— Start at 5 mcg/kg/min

Special Considerations

— 10% of patient's weight (in lbs) is roughly the drops per minute for 5 mcg/kg/min.

— Ex: 120 lbs patient at 5 mcg/kg/min is about 12 drops per minute (exact = 10.2 gtts/min)

— Use 60 gtts tubing (pediatric) tubing

EPINEPHRINE

Name(s): Adrenalin

Class: sympathomimetic

MOA

— alpha: peripheral vasoconstriction beta$_1$: positive inotrope, chronotrope, dromotrope beta$_2$: bronchodilator

— Clinical effects: increased cerebral & myocardial perfusion, increases HR, BP & myocardial electrical activity, reverses bronchospasm, anaphylaxis

Packaging

— 1:10,000: 1 mg/10 mL prefilled syringe

— 1:1,000: 1 mg/1 mL amp & 30mg/30mL multi-dose vial

Indications

— Cardiac arrest: all causes

— Severe bronchospasm

— Anaphylaxis

— Symptomatic bradycardia (not first line)

— Hypotension (non-hypovolemic causes)

Contraindications

— None for cardiac arrest

— Hypothermia (relative)

Adverse Reactions

— CV: hypertension, dysrhythmia, tachycardia, angina

— CNS: agitation, anxiety

— GI: N&V

Adult Dose: cardiac arrest

— IV: 1 mg 1:10,000 q 3–5 min. followed by 20 mL flush. No max dose.

— ETT: 2–2.5 mg of 1:1,000 diluted to 10 mL

Adult Dose: hypotension, bradycardia

— 2–10 mcg/min infusion titrate to effect.

— Add 1 mg epi to 250 mL = 4 mcg/mL

Adult Dose: asthma, anaphylaxis

— 0.3–0.5 mg 1:1,000 IM preferred (can also administer SC or inject SL)

Peds Dose

— IV/IO initial dose for cardiac arrest or refractory bradycardia: 0.01 mg/kg of 1:10,000 (0.1 mL/kg)

— ET initial dose for cardiac arrest or refractory bradycardia: 0.1 mg/kg of 1:1,000 diluted with NS to 3–5 mL (0.1 mL/kg)

Special Considerations

— For epi infusion, 1 mg epi in 250 mL = 4 mcg per mL

— Admin 15 drops per min for every mcg per min. Ex:

  • 1 mcg/min = 15 gtts/min

  • 2 mcg/min = 30 gtts/min

FENTANYL

Name(s): Actiq, Duragesic, Sublimaze

Class: Narcotic analgesic (synthetic)

MOA: CNS depression, pain reliever, decreased preload and afterload

Packaging
— 100 mcg/2 mL or
— 250 mcg/5 mL
— Note: both are 50 mcg/mL

Indications
— Analgesia (burns, trauma, MI, renal colic)
— Sedation
— RSI or med-assisted intubation

Contraindications
— Known allergy
— Respiratory depression
— Increased ICP
— Hypotension
— Head injury with ALOC (relative)
— Asthma (relative)
— Abdominal pain (relative)

Adverse Reactions
— MS: muscle rigidity (often chest)
— CV: dysrhythmias, hypotension
— Resp: resp. depression
— CNS: excess sedation, seizures, coma
— GI: N&V

Adult Dose
— IV/IO: 25–50 mcg slow IVP (1–5 min)
— IM: same as IV/IO (slower onset)
— Notes:
  • Total dose NOT to exceed 200 mcg
  • Resp dep may last longer than analgesic

Peds Dose: 1–2 mcg/kg (max 50 mcg)

Special Considerations
— Caution: 50–100 times more powerful than morphine
— Do NOT administer more than 50 mcg (1 mL) in a single dose

GLUCAGON

Name(s): Glucagon

Class: Pancreatic hormone, hyperglycemic agent

MOA: Converts glycogen to glucose, counteracts insulin

Packaging: 1 mg/1mL vials (reconstitution required)

Indications: Symptomatic hypoglycemia when IV access is delayed

Contraindications: Known allergy

Adverse Reactions: N&V (rare)

Dose:

— Adult (over 44 lbs/20kg: 1 mg IM

— Peds: 0.5 mg IM

IPRATROPIUM BROMIDE

Name(s): Atrovent

Class: Anticholinergic, bronchodilator

MOA: Inhibits parasympathetic NS, preferential dilation of larger central airways

Packaging: 500 mcg/2.5 mL unit dose

Indications

— Bronchospasm

— Can be used alone or combined with albuterol

Contraindications

— Known allergy

— Allergy to atropine

— Caution in patients with angle closure glaucoma

Adverse Reactions

— Resp: cough, increased sputum production

— CNS: dizziness, insomnia, tremors, nervousness

— GI: nausea

Adult Dose:

— 500 mcg in 2.5 mL unit dose via SVN or in-line with BVM

— Can be mixed with albuterol

LIDOCAINE

Name(s): Xylocaine

Class: Antidysrhythmic, local anesthetic

MOA: Increases VF threshold, decrease ventricular irritability

Packaging

— 100 mg/5 mL prefilled syringe (20 mg per mL)

— 1 g/25 mL vial (must be added to 250 mL) *OR*

— 2 g/500 mL premix bag

Indications

— VT, VF, pulseless VT (amiodarone preferred)

— Maintenance infusion after conversion from VT, VF

— Frequent PVCs (above 6/min, 2 or more consecutive PVCs, multiform PVCs, R-on-T PVCs)

Contraindications

— Known allergy

— 2nd or 3rd degree block

— Do NOT use if heart rate below 60 (treat bradycardia first)

Adverse Reactions

— Drowsiness

— Bradycardia

— Paresthesia

— Tinnitus

— Seizures

Adult Dose: VF, pulseless VT

— Initial bolus of 1–1.5 mg/kg IVP

— Repeat if needed q 5–10 min. at 0.5 to 0.75 mg/kg to max of 3 mg/kg

Adult Dose: vent. ectopy with a pulse

— Initial bolus of 0.5 to 1.5 mg/kg IVP

— Repeat at 0.5–0.75 mg/kg if needed q 5–10 min. to max dose of 3 mg/kg

Adult Dose: maintenance infusion

— Infuse 2–4 mg/min (total mg/kg dose + 1)

— Prepare solution with 1 gram in 250 mL NS or 2 grams in 500 mL NS for concentration of 4 mg/mL

— Pts over 70 or with hepatic, renal disease, poor perfusion, CHF: cut maintenance infusion in half

Special Considerations

— To quickly determine mL for bolus: cut total dose in half and move decimal to left. Ex: 60 mg = 3 mL

— Infusion = 15 gtts per min for every mg per min (use 60 gtts tubing)

- 1 mg/min = 15 gtts/min
- 2 mg/min = 30 gtts/min
- 3 mg/min = 45 gtts/min
- 4 mg/min = 60 gtts/min

LORAZEPAM

Name(s): Ativan

Class: Benzodiazepine

MOA: CNS depression, anti-convulsant

Packaging

— 2 mg/mL or

— 4 mg/mL

Indications

— Seizures, status epilepticus

— Agitated (excited) delirium

Contraindications

— Known allergy

— Acute angle closure glaucoma

— Myasthenia gravis

— Pregnancy (relative)

Adverse Reactions
- — Confusion
- — Sedation
- — Amnesia
- — Hypotension
- — Respiratory depression

Adult Dose
- — Seizures: 2–5 mg slow IV/IO (at least 2 min). Max 10 mg
- — Note: may be given deep IM if no IV/IO access

Peds Dose
- — Seizures: 0.05–0.1 mg/kg slow IV/IO (at least 2 min) max 4 mg
- — Note: may be given deep IM if no IV/IO access

MAGNESIUM SULFATE

Name(s): Magnesium sulfate, $MgSO_4$

Class: Electrolyte, tocolytic, antidysrhythmic

MOA: Decrease ventricular irritability, inhibits muscular excitability

Packaging: 1 g/2 mL vials

Indications
- — Polymorphic V-tach
- — VF/Pulseless VT refractory to amiodarone or lido
- — Hypomagnesemia
- — Pre-term labor
- — Pregnancy-induced hypertension (pre-eclampsia and eclampsia)

Contraindications
- — Known allergy
- — Heart block
- — Hypermagnesemia
- — Severe renal impairment

Adverse Reactions
- — CV: hypotension, dysrhythmias
- — Resp: resp. depression or paralysis
- — CNS: sweaty, drowsy, depressed reflexes

— GI: nausea

— Other: flushed

— Note: calcium may help reverse MgSO$_4$ toxicity

Adult Dose: cardiac arrest

— VF/pulseless VT: 1–2 grams IV over 1–2 min

— Polymorphic VT: 1–2 grams IV over 1–2 min followed by 1–2 grams over 1 hour

— Note: if resp. rate drops below 12 per min, discontinue MgSO$_4$

Adult Dose: OB

— Pre-term labor/Pre-eclampsia/Eclampsia: 4 grams in 100 mL over 15 min.

— Note: if resp. rate drops below 12 per min, discontinue MgSO$_4$

MIDAZOLAM

Name(s): Versed

Class: Benzodiazepine

MOA: CNS depression, anti-convulsant, sedation

Packaging: 5 mg/5 mL vial

Indications

— Anticonvulsant

— Sedation

— Facilitation of intubation

— Acute agitation/excited delirium

Contraindications

— Known allergy

— Angle closure glaucoma

— Neuromuscular disorders (relative)

— Intoxication (relative)

— COPD (relative)

— Resp compromise (relative)

— Pregnancy (relative)

Adverse Reactions

— CV: cardiac arrest, dysrhythmias, hypotension

— Resp: resp. depression, wheezing, coughing, hiccups

— CNS: tremors, drowsiness, headache

— GI: N&V

— Note: resp arrest possible when used with narcotics or if administered too rapidly

Adult Dose

— Sedation: patients 14–60 years of age:

  • 1–10 mg slow IV/IO titrate to effect (max 2.5 mg over 2 min)

  • 2–5 mg IM

— Sedation: patients over 60 years of age:

  • 1–3.5 mg slow IV/IO as above

  • 1–5 mg IM

— Seizures (no IV/IO access): 0.2 mg/kg deep IM

Peds Dose

— IV/IO: 0.05–0.1 mg/kg slow push

— IM/IN: 0.2 mg/kg if no IV/IO access

MORPHINE

Name(s): Morphine

Class: Narcotic analgesic

MOA: CNS depression, pain reliever, decreased preload and afterload

Packaging: 10 mg 1 mL ampule or syringe

Indications

— Analgesia (burns, trauma, MI, renal colic)

— Cardiogenic pulmonary edema

Contraindications

— Known allergy

— Respiratory depression

— Hypovolemia

— Hypotension

— Head injury

— Increased ICP

— Asthma (relative)

— Abdominal pain (relative)

Adverse Reactions

— CV: bradycardia, orthostatic hypotension

— Resp: resp depression

— CNS: seizures, coma

— GI: N&V

Adult Dose: 1–3 mg slow IVP titrate to effect

NALOXONE

Name(s): Narcan

Class: Narcotic antagonist

MOA: Competitively blocks narcotic receptor sites, reverses respiratory depression due to narcotics

Packaging: 0.4 mg ampules & 1 mg/mL prefilled syringe

Indications

— Narcotic overdose

— Unconscious patient of unknown etiology

Contraindications: Known allergy

Adverse Reactions

— May not reverse histamine effects of narcotic OD

— Withdrawal symptoms

— Combative patient

— Shorter half-life than many narcotics (risk of secondary overdose)

Adult Dose

— IV, ET, IM, SQ, SL: 2 mg as needed, titrate to effect

— Intra-nasal: 1 mg each nostril with Mucosal Atomizer Device, repeat as needed

— Note: may substitute with nalmefene (Revex) 2 mg

Peds Dose: Under 5 years of age: 0.1 mg/kg IV, ET, SL, SC, IO

NITROGLYCERINE

Name(s): Nitrostat, Tridil

Class: Vasodilator, organic nitrate, antianginal

MOA: Decreased preload & afterload, coronary artery vasodilation, increased myocardial oxygen supply, decreased myocardial oxygen demand

Packaging: 0.4 mg tablets or spray

Indications

— Angina

— MI

— CHF with pulmonary edema

Contraindications

— Hypotension

— Hypovolemia

— Increased ICP

— Erectile dysfunction meds (Ex: Viagra, Levitra, Cialis)

Adverse Reactions

— Hypotension

— Reflex tachycardia

— Headache

— Burning under tongue

Adult Dose

— 0.4 mg tablet or spray

— May repeat × 3 with BP over 100 systolic & medical direction approval

— Establish IV access prior to administration

NITROUS OXIDE

Name(s): Nitronox

Class: Inhaled analgesic

MOA: CNS depression, pain reliever

Packaging: 50–50 oxygen/nitrous oxide mix

Indications: Temporary pain relief from musculoskeletal trauma, burns

Contraindications

— Unconscious patient

— Respiratory compromise, pneumothorax

— Abdominal pain

— Head injury

Adverse Reactions

— Resp: worsening of pneumothorax

— GI: N&V, intestinal rupture

Adult Dose: Inhaled, self-administered

OXYGEN

Name: Oxygen (O_2)

Class: Gas

MOA: Increases tissue oxygenation

Packaging: 50–50 oxygen/nitrous oxide mix

Indications

— Cardiac arrest

— Bradycardia in infants/peds

— Any patient receiving PPV

— Suspected hypoxia, shock, TBI

— SpO_2 below 94%

Contraindications: Unsafe conditions

Adverse Reactions

— Hyperoxia

— Possible resp depression in COPD patients

Dose: Sufficient to maintain SpO_2 of at least 94%

OXYTOCIN

Name(s): Pitocin, Syntocin

Class: Hormone, uterine stimulant

MOA: Increases force and frequency of uterine contractions

Packaging: 10 units/1 mL ampule or vial

Indications: Severe postpartum hemorrhage (over 500 mL) within first 24 hrs

Contraindications: Known allergy

Adverse Reactions

— CV: shock, tachycardia

— Resp: anaphylaxis

— GI: N&V

Adult Dose

— 10–20 units in 1,000 mL NS or LR titrate to effect

— Can also administer 10 units IM

— Note: use only after delivery of the placenta

PROMETHAZINE

Name(s): Phenergan

Class: Antiemetic, antihistamine

MOA: Blocks histamine receptors

Packaging

— 25 mg/1 mL vial

— 50 mg/1 mL vial

Indications

— N&V

— Sedation

Contraindications: Known allergy to Phenergan, Compazine, Thorazine

Adverse Reactions

— Extravasation can cause tissue necrosis

— May lower seizure threshold

— Sedation, drowsiness

— Extrapyramidal symptoms

Adult Dose: N&V

— 12.5 mg IV or deep IM (NOT SQ!)

— Older patients: 6.25 mg

— Not for children under 2 years old

— Children over 2 years: consult medical direction

— Note: Ondansetron (Zofran) often preferred due to limited side effects and contraindications

THIAMINE

Name(s): Vit. B_1, Betalin

Class: Vitamin

MOA: Required for carbohydrate metabolism

Packaging: 100 mg/1 mL ampule or tubex

Indications

— Alcoholism, delirium tremens

— Coma of unknown etiology

— Wernicke-Korsakoff syndrome (thiamine deficiency)

Contraindications: None

Adverse Reactions: Hypotension (rare)

Adult Dose: 100 mg IV or IM

VII. ADDITIONAL PARAMEDIC MEDICATIONS

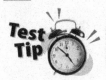

The following medications are not listed as "must know" in the NEMSES. However, they are utilized by paramedics in many areas. These medications are not likely to be tested on the national certification exam.

BUMETANIDE

Name(s): Bumex

Class and MOA: Loop diuretic

Indications

— Pulmonary edema

— CHF

Contraindications

— Known allergy to drug or sulfa drugs

— Anuria

— Dehydration

Adverse Reactions

— Dizzy

— Headache

— Hypotension

— Cardiac dysrhythmia

— N&V

— Tinnitus

CALCIUM

Class and MOA

— Electrolyte

— Positive inotrope

Indications

— Acute hypocalcemia

— Acute hyperkalemia

— Ca channel blocker OD

— Pretreatment for verapamil or diltiazem

Contraindications

— Hypercalcemia

— Concurrent digoxin therapy (relative)

Adverse Reactions

— Asystole

— Bradycardia

— Tissue necrosis on infiltration

— Cardiac dysrhythmias if taking digoxin

DEXAMETHASONE

Name(s): Decadron

Class and MOA

— Glucocorticoid

— Anti-inflammatory

Indications

— Reactive airway disease

— Asthma

— Anaphylaxis

Contraindications

— Known allergy

— Allergy to sulfa drugs

Adverse Reactions

— Edema

— Hypertension

— Convulsions

— Anaphylaxis

FUROSEMIDE

Name(s): Lasix

Class and MOA

— Loop diuretic

— Vasodilation

— Diuresis

Indications

— Pulmonary edema

— CHF

Contraindications

— Hypersensitivity (to Lasix or sulfa drugs)

— Hypotension

— Hypovolemia

Adverse Reactions

— Anuria

— Hypokalemia

— Hyperglycemia

— Hypovolemia

METHYLPREDNISOLONE

Name(s): Solu-Medrol

Class and MOA

— Steroid

— Anti-inflammatory

— Stabilizes cell membrane

Indications

— Reactive airway disease

— Anaphylaxis

— Airway burns

Contraindications: Hypersensitivity

Adverse Reactions: None from single dose

NALMEFENE

Name(s): Revex

Class and MOA

— Narcotic antagonist

— Competitively inhibits narcotic receptor sites

Indications: Suspected narcotic overdose

Contraindications: Hypersensitivity

Adverse Reactions

— Withdrawal symptoms

— N&V

— Pulmonary edema

— Dysrhythmias

— Combative

ONDANSETRON

Name(s): Zofran

Class and MOA: Anti-emetic

Indications: N&V

Contraindications

— Hypersensitivity

— Long QT syndrome

— Caution in patients w/ liver problems

Adverse Reactions

— Headache

— Fatigue

— Diarrhea

PHENYLEPHRINE

Name(s): Neo-Synephrine

Class and MOA: Topical vasoconstrictor

Indications: Reduce bleeding during nasal intubation

Contraindications: Hypersensitivity

Adverse Reactions: None

SODIUM BICARB

Class and MOA
— Buffer
— Raises pH

Indications
— Metabolic acidosis
— Aspirin or cyclic antidepressant OD
— Cardiac arrest (last line)

Contraindications: Alkalosis

Adverse Reactions
— CHF
— Edema
— Intracellular acidosis
— Tissue necrosis on infiltration

SUCCINYLCHOLINE

Name(s): Anectine, Quelicin

Class and MOA
— Short acting neuromuscular blocker
— Paralytic

Indications: Facilitation of rapid sequence induction (RSI)

Contraindications
— Hypersensitivity
— Hyperkalemia
— Malignant hyperthermia
— Penetrating eye injuries
— Airway obstruction
— Neuromuscular disorder
— Epiglottitis
— Burns, crush injury

Adverse Reactions
— Prolonged apnea

— Fasciculations

— Hyperkalemia

— Inability to intubate following paralysis

VERAPAMIL

Name(s): Isoptin, Calan, Verelan

Class and MOA
— Calcium channel blocker

— Negative inotrope

— Slows AV conduction

Indications
— SVT (not first-line drug)

— a-fib, a-flutter with rapid vent response

Contraindications
— Hypersensitivity

— 2nd or 3rd degree AV block

— Sick sinus syndrome

— Wide QRS tachy

— Shock, CHF

— WPW syndrome

Adverse Reactions
— Extreme bradycardia

— Hypotension

— Heart block

— Asystole

— CHF

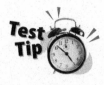

Patient assessment should be thought of as the 7th category on the national certification exam. The exam will be full of questions that challenge your patient assessment skills. These are often scenario-based questions. Thoroughly memorize the components of patient assessment from scene size-up through reassessment. Knowing the order of the steps and priorities for patient assessment will help guide you to the correct answer.

PART II

AIRWAY/ASSESSMENT/ BLEEDING AND SHOCK

Airway, Oxygenation, Ventilation

TERMS TO KNOW

A. Cellular respiration—cellular processes that convert energy from nutrients into adenosine triphosphate (ATP), and then release waste products

B. Exhalation—the passive part of breathing

C. External respiration—oxygen exchange between the lungs and circulatory system

D. Hypoxia—oxygen deficiency

E. Inhalation—the active part of breathing

F. Internal respiration—oxygen exchange between blood and cells of the body

G. Minute ventilation—volume of gas inhaled or exhaled per minute (respiratory rate x tidal volume)

H. Oxygenation—delivery of oxygen to the blood

I. Ventilation—the physical movement of moving air in and out of the lungs

II. ANATOMY AND PHYSIOLOGY REVIEW

A. Airway structures

1. Upper airway

   i.   Nose and mouth

   ii. Nasopharynx, oropharynx

   > **Note:** The oropharynx houses the tongue (primary cause of upper airway obstruction in unresponsive patients).

   iii. Epiglottis

   iv. Larynx (the portion above the vocal cords)

2. Lower airway

   i.   Larynx (the portion below the vocal cords)

   ii. Trachea

   iii. Left and right mainstem bronchi

   iv. Bronchioles

   v.   Alveoli

   > **Note:** The alveoli are the "terminal" (end) structure in the lower airway.

B. Regulation of ventilation

1. Hypoxia

   i.   Early signs and symptoms of hypoxia

   ➤ Restless, anxious, irritable

   ➤ Tachycardia and tachypnea

   ii. Late signs and symptoms of hypoxia

   ➤ Decreased LOC

   ➤ Severe dyspnea

➤ Cyanosis

➤ Bradycardia (especially in pediatric patients)

2. CO_2 drive

  i. The primary system for monitoring breathing status.

  ii. Monitors CO_2 levels in blood and cerebrospinal fluid.

  iii. Chemoreceptors in brainstem detect increased CO_2 and rapidly trigger increased respiratory rate.

3. Hypoxic drive

  i. Backup system to CO_2 drive

  ii. Monitors oxygen levels in plasma.

  iii. May be present in end-stage COPD patients.

  iv. Prolonged exposure to high concentration oxygen in hypoxic drive patients can cause respiratory depression.

4. Acid-base disorders

  i. Four primary acid-base disorders can affect regulation of ventilation.

    ➤ Primary respiratory problems

      — Respiratory acidosis: Look for blood gas with low pH and elevated CO_2.

      — Respiratory alkalosis: Look for blood gas with elevated pH and low CO_2.

Note: A primary respiratory problem presents with $PaCO_2$ less than 35 mmHg (alkalosis) or greater than 45 mmHg (acidosis).

    ➤ Primary metabolic problems

      — Metabolic acidosis: Look for blood gas with low pH and low HCO_3 level.

      — Metabolic alkalosis: Look for elevated pH and elevated HCO_3 level.

Note: A primary metabolic problem presents with HCO_3 below 22 mmHg (acidosis) or greater than 26mmHg (alkalosis).

    ii. Normal arterial blood gas values

➤ pH: 7.35–7.45

➤ PaO_2: 80–100 mmHg

➤ $PaCO_2$: 35–45 mmHg

➤ HCO_3: 22–26 mEq/L

➤ SaO_2: 95% or above

C. Oxygenation

1. Effective ventilation is required for adequate oxygenation.

2. Adequate oxygenation is required for effective respiration.

3. Adequate oxygenation does *not* ensure effective internal respiration.

4. Ventilation does *not* ensure oxygenation (e.g., ventilation can occur without oxygenation during smoke inhalation or CO poisoning).

5. Delivering supplemental oxygen can only improve cellular oxygenation if ventilations are adequate and result in external and internal respiration.

D. Respiration

1. Effective respiration results in cellular exchange of O_2 and CO_2.

2. Time and injury

    i. Without adequate respiration:

➤ Heart and brain become irritable almost immediately

➤ Brain damage likely within 4 minutes

➤ Permanent brain damage likely within 6 minutes

➤ Irrecoverable brain damage (biological death) likely within 10 minutes

E. Ventilation-perfusion mismatch

1. aka V/Q mismatch or V/Q defect

2. Occurs when the lungs receive oxygen, but not adequate blood flow *or* when the lungs receive blood flow, but inadequate oxygen.

3. V/Q mismatch could begin as either a ventilatory (oxygenation & respiration) problem or a perfusion problem, e.g., pulmonary embolism.

III. AIRWAY

A. Manual airway techniques come first (as indicated).

1. Head-tilt, chin lift (preferred)

2. Jaw-thrust (suspected spinal injury)

B. Suction (as indicated) comes second.

1. Rigid suction catheters

   i. Used to suction oral airway

   ii. aka tonsil tip or Yankauer catheter

2. French suction catheters

   i. Used to suction nose, stoma, or inside advanced airway.

   ii. aka soft-tip, whistle-tip or flexible catheter

   iii. Available in numerous sizes (diameters) (e.g., 3 French through 40 French. Increased number = increased diameter)

3. Suction time cannot exceed:

   i. 15 seconds for adults

   ii. 10 seconds for pediatrics

   iii. 5 seconds for infants

C. Mechanical airway adjuncts come third (as indicated).

1. Basic adjuncts

   i. OPA: for unresponsive patients without a gag reflect (avoid posterior displacement of tongue)

   ii. NPA: can be used on patients with decreased LOC, but not unresponsive

2. Advanced airway management

   i. Extraglottic, retroglottic and supraglottic airway devices

      ➤ Common types used prehospital

         — Laryngeal Mask Airway (LMA) and LMA Supreme

         — i-gel supraglottic LMA

         — Pharyngeal Tracheal Lumen Airway (PTL)

         — Esophageal Tracheal Combitube (ETC)

         — King LT Airway

         — Supraglottic Airway Laryngopharyngeal Tube (SALT)

      ➤ Advantages

         — Easy to use

         — Blind insertion, no laryngoscope needed

         — Able to insert quickly

         — High success rate (avoid posterior displacement of tongue)

   ii. Endotracheal intubation (ETT)

      ➤ Advantages

         — Isolates the trachea

         — Eliminates gastric distention from ventilation

         — No mask seal needed

         — Improved suctioning ability

         — Route for medication administration (naloxone, epinephrine, atropine, lidocaine)

      ➤ Disadvantages

         — Extensive training required

         — Direct visualization of vocal cords required

         — Takes longer than other advanced airways

         — Has many serious complications

         — Not been shown to increase survival rates

> Verification of proper ETT placement

— Direct visualization of cords

— Auscultation of epigastrium and bilateral lung fields

— Continuous waveform capnography

— Pulse oximetry

— Esophageal detector device

— ETT introducer

iii. Surgical cricothyrotomy

> Only indicated in acute, life-threatening situations when use of less invasive airway techniques are ineffective.

iv. Rapid sequence induction (intubation) or medication-assisted intubation

> Indications

— Respiratory failure

— Inability to protect airway

— Combative patient, suspected TBI

— Persistent hypoxia

> Contraindications

— Respiratory and cardiac arrest

— Anticipated difficult airway (relative)

— Short transport time (relative)

— Ability to manage airway with less invasive measures

— Neuromuscular disease, e.g., ALS, muscular dystrophy

v. Predictors of difficult advanced airway insertion

> Mouth does not fully open

> Hypersecretions

> Obesity

> Pulmonary edema

> Airway burns

> Facial trauma

➤ Increased Mallampati score (used with oral intubation)

— Class I: entire tonsil clear

— Class II: upper half of tonsil visible

— Class III: soft and hard palate visible

— Class IV: only hard palate visible

➤ LEMONS mnemonic for difficult airway

— L: look externally

— E: evaluate 3–3–2 rule

— M: Mallampati score

— O: obstruction

— N: neck mobility

— S: saturations

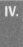 IV. OXYGENATION

A. Indications for supplemental oxygen

1. Dyspnea

2. Hypoxia

3. Pulse oximeter below 94%

4. Altered or decreased LOC

5. Respiratory or cardiac arrest

6. Hypoperfusion (shock)

B. Supplemental oxygen devices

1. Nasal cannula

i. Low-flow oxygen

ii. Up to 6 lpm can be administered

iii. Delivers 24%–44% oxygen (about 4% per liter above 21% room air)

2. Non-rebreather

    i.   High-flow oxygen

    ii. 12–15 lpm

    iii. Delivers about 90% oxygen

3. Small volume nebulizer (SVN)

    i.   Used for delivery of aerosolized medication

C. Oxygen cylinders

1. Cylinder sizes

    i.   D cylinder: about 350-liter capacity

    ii. E cylinder: about 625-liter capacity

    iii. M cylinder: about 3,000-liter capacity

2. Oxygen cylinder pressure

    i.   Full cylinder is about 2,000 PSI

    ii. Safe residual pressure is 200 PSI (Cylinder should be taken out of service and refilled once it reaches 200 PSI.)

D. Pin indexing system

1. Safety feature that prevents an oxygen regulator from being connected to a tank with any other compressed gas (e.g., CO_2 tank).

E. Calculating duration of an oxygen tank

1. Formula:

$$\frac{(\text{cylinder PSI} - \text{safe residual pressure}) \times \text{tank constant}}{\text{remaining flow rate (lpm)}} = \text{minutes}$$

2. Tank constants:

    i.   D cylinder constant: 0.16

    ii. E cylinder constant: 0.28

    iii. M cylinder constant: 1.56

Example: You are administering 15 lpm via NRB with a D cylinder oxygen tank with 1,500 PSI remaining.
(1,300 x 0.16) ÷ 15 = 13.86 minutes

V. **VENTILATION**

A. Initiate PPV for any patient with signs of inadequate breathing, such as:

1. Excessively bradypneic or tachypneic breathing (age-dependent)

2. Shallow breathing

3. Altered or decreased LOC

4. Dyspnea

5. Retractions

6. Accessory muscle use

7. Cyanosis

8. Paradoxical motion

9. Sucking chest wound

B. When in doubt, ventilate. (Patients that don't need it will let you know.)

C. Rates of ventilation

1. Do *not* hyperventilate It increases the risk of gastric distention, vomiting, aspiration, ineffective CPR, and death

    i. Adults: ventilate at 10–12 breaths per minute

    ii. Children and infants: ventilate at 12–20 breaths per minute

D. Tidal volumes during PPV

1. Rise and fall of the chest is an indication of adequate ventilation.

2. It should take about 1 second to inflate the chest during PPV.

E. Complications of PPV

1. Increased intrathoracic pressure and reduced cardiac output

2. Gastric distention and increased risk of vomiting

> **Note:** Use of the Sellick technique (cricoid pressure) to reduce gastric distention is not recommended and should never be used during active vomiting.

F. Automatic transport ventilators (ATVs)

 1. ATVs allow for automated PPV with set rates and tidal volumes.

 2. Tidal volume based on 6–7 mL/kg of ideal body weight

 3. Advantages

  i. Very consistent rates and tidal volumes

  ii. May reduce risk of hyperventilation

  iii. Allows for hand-free ventilation if advanced airway in place

 4. Disadvantages

  i. Unable to assess BVM compliance

  ii. Must base tidal volume on ideal body weight, or risk pulmonary overpressurization of obese patients

  iii. Pressure relief valve may prevent effective ventilation in patients requiring higher pressures. (Disable as indicated.)

 ## VI. BREATHING PATTERNS

A. Agonal respirations—Slow, shallow, infrequent breaths; indicates brain anoxia.

B. Biot's respirations—Irregular pattern of rate and depth and periodic apnea; indicates increased ICP.

C. Central neurologic hyperventilation—Deep, rapid respirations; indicates increased ICP.

D. Cheyne-Stokes respirations—Progressively deeper and faster breaths, changing to slower and shallow breaths; indicates brain injury.

E. Kussmaul respirations—Deep, gasping breaths; indicates possible DKA.

VII. BREATH SOUNDS

A. Rales (crackles)—Fine, bubbling sound on inspiration; indicates fluid in lower airways.

B. Rhonchi—Course sounds on inspiration; indicates inflammation or mucus in lower airways.

C. Wheezes—High-pitched sound on inspiration or expiration; indicates bronchoconstriction.

D. Snoring—Indicates partial airway obstruction from the tongue.

E. Stridor—High-pitched sound indicating significant upper airway obstruction (e.g., foreign body, angioedema, anaphylaxis)

F. Gurgling—Indicates fluid in the upper airway.

 VIII. PATIENT MONITORING TECHNOLOGY

A. Pulse oximetry (SpO_2)

   1. Measures oxygenation.

   2. Can take several minutes to see changes in oxygenation (use with continuous waveform capnography if available).

   3. Can also be used to monitor pulse rate (visual and/or auditory).

   4. Should be used with capnography when possible.

B. Capnography ($ETCO_2$)

   1. Measures carbon dioxide and ventilatory status.

   2. Reflects changes in ventilatory status almost immediately.

   3. Should be used with pulse oximetry when possible.

   4. Types of capnography

      i. Capnometry—provides a numeric display of expired CO_2

      ii. Capnography—graphic display of capnometry

      iii. Colorimetric $ETCO_2$—disposable color changing device placed between the patient and the ventilation device

   5. Normal arterial CO_2 ($PaCO_2$) and $ETCO_2$ values are about 35–45 mmHg.

   6. Clinical application of capnography

      i. High $ETCO_2$—possible hypoventilation

      ii. Low $ETCO_2$—possible hyperventilation

      iii. $ETCO_2$ drops to 0 — possible for esophageal intubation or displaced tube

      iv. Sharp drop in $ETCO_2$ — possible pulmonary embolism, cardiac arrest, hypotension, hyperventilation

C. Pulse CO oximetry

  1. Newer technology available in prehospital that can detect carboxyhemoglobin and methemoglobin.

IX. CONTINUOUS POSITIVE AIRWAY PRESSURE (CPAP)

A. Indications

  1. Indicated for alert and spontaneously breathing patients, at least 12 years of age, in significant respiratory distress, such as sleep apnea, COPD, pulmonary edema, CHF, pneumonia.

  2. Candidates for CPAP should demonstrate significant distress, such as tachypnea, SpO_2 below 94%, and/or use of accessory muscles.

  3. Typical starting range 5–7 cm H_2O

B. Contraindications

  1. Apnea

  2. Patients unable to follow verbal commands

  3. Suspected pneumothorax

  4. Chest trauma

  5. Tracheostomy

  6. Vomiting

  7. GI bleeding

  8. Hypotension

X. SPECIAL SITUATIONS

A. Pediatric patients

  1. Pediatric airway more easily obstructed.

  2. Place padding behind shoulders of supine patient to align airway.

3. Do not overextend the head and neck during head-tilt, chin-lift.

4. Reduce tidal volume to avoid hyperventilation, gastric distention, or pulmonary over pressurization.

5. Hypoxia develops quickly.

6. Hypoxia is the most common cause of bradycardia in peds.

7. Always assume hypoxia in a bradycardic peds patient.

B. Tracheostomy tube/stoma

1. BVM will connect directly to trach tube.

2. To ventilate a patient with stoma (no trach tube) use an infant or peds mask with appropriate-size BVM. Seal mouth and nose during ventilation.

3. Trach tubes and stomas require frequent suctioning.

C. Dentures

1. Dentures are usually secured in place and can be left alone.

2. If dentures are loose and interfere with airway management or ventilations, they should be removed.

D. Foreign body airway obstruction (FBAO)

1. BLS

   i. Conscious adults and children (not infants): abdominal thrusts

   ii. Unconscious (all ages): chest compressions

   iii. Conscious infants: back blows and chest thrusts

2. ALS (when BLS interventions are ineffective)

   i. Attempt to remove foreign body with laryngoscope and McGill forceps.

   ii. Attempt ETT insertion to try passing tube through obstruction or forcing it into right mainstem.

E. Stridor (suspected croup or epiglottitis)

1. Keep patient calm.

2. Use supplemental oxygen if pulse ox below 95%.

3. Consider saline SVN or nebulized epinephrine (per local protocol).

4. Avoid aggressive airway interventions unless airway becomes completely obstructed.

F. Respiratory burns

1. Consider rapid intubation for patients with airway burns due to risk of massive swelling (whatever degree of airway swelling apparent on initial contact will almost certainly get worse).

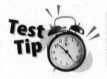

When you get patient care scenarios on the certification exam, don't hesitate to ventilate! If you are unsure if you should ventilate your patient, and ventilation is an option, then you probably should.

Patient Assessment

I. TERMS TO KNOW

A. Ascites—abdominal swelling (consider liver disease, CHF, renal failure)

B. Cullen's sign—bruising around the umbilicus (consider intra-abdominal bleeding)

C. Field impression—A field conclusion of the patient's problem based on the clinical presentation and the exclusion of other possible causes through considering the differential diagnoses.

D. Grey Turner's sign—bruising over flanks (consider intra-abdominal bleeding)

E. Pitting edema—depression left by pressure of finger (consider CHF, renal failure)

II. OVERVIEW OF PATIENT ASSESSMENT

A. The 5 major components of patient assessment:

1. Scene size-up

2. Primary assessment

3. Patient history

4. Secondary assessment

5. Reassessment

B. Patient assessment tips

1. Patient assessment in the field is not always linear, and you may not get to every component on every patient; however, it helps to think of it in a linear format as follows:

   i. The scene size-up always comes first and continues throughout the call.

   ii. The primary assessment comes next and precedes all other components of patient assessment.

   iii. The order and priority of the patient history and secondary assessment can change based on the patient's complaint and condition.

   iv. Reassessment is the final step in the assessment process.

2. Significant trauma patients tend to demand a more intensive primary and secondary assessment and the secondary assessment would take priority over the patient history.

3. Conscious medical patients often demand a more thorough patient history than some trauma patients, and the patient history would take a higher priority than the secondary assessment.

4. The NREMT skill sheets for trauma assessment and medical assessment hint at the above concepts. Look at how many points are awarded for the secondary assessment and the patient history on both skill sheets.

5. Regardless of the patient's complaint, the patient assessment must be organized and methodical.

C. Forming a field impression

1. Differential diagnosis based on history and physical exam

2. Consider past experience

3. Gut instinct (sick/not sick)

 III. **SCENE SIZE-UP**

A. Scene safety

B. Standard precautions

C. Mechanism of injury (c-spine indicated?) or nature of illness (medical patients)

D. Number of patients

E. Additional resources

IV. PRIMARY ASSESSMENT

A. Primary assessment tips:

1. The primary assessment begins as soon as you locate the patient.

2. The purpose of the primary assessment is to find and manage immediately life-threatening conditions.

3. The primary assessment may take only seconds in a conscious, stable patient or you may not be able to move past the primary assessment in a patient with ongoing life threats.

4. Components of the primary assessment:

   i. General impression

   ii. Spinal precautions and expose patient as indicated

   iii. Level of consciousness (AVPU)

   iv. ABCs (or CAB, if patient unresponsive)

     ➤ Airway

       — Manual, suction, mechanical

       — BLS before ALS

     ➤ Breathing

       — Support ventilations and provide supplemental oxygen as indicated.

       — Manage flail chest (with PPV) and sucking chest wounds (with occlusive dressing) as indicated.

     ➤ Circulation

       — Assess pulse, CPR as indicated.

— Manage life-threatening bleeding.

    (i) Direct pressure

    (ii) Tourniquet

    (iii) Hemostatic agent if tourniquet not possible (e.g., torso)

— Assess circulation to skin (color, temp, moisture).

v. Rapid scan aka rapid secondary (as indicated)

➤ Indicated for unresponsive patients, significant trauma patients, or any patient suspected of having additional life-threatening injuries (e.g., internal bleeding, unstable pelvis, femur fracture, etc.).

➤ Note that some sources regard the rapid scan as a late component of the primary assessment while others consider it the beginning of the secondary assessment. This is largely irrelevant as it bridges the two components of assessment either way.

➤ The rapid scan is used to identify any remaining life threats and should not take longer than about 90 seconds. Do *not* spend time on non-life-threatening conditions during the rapid scan.

➤ The rapid scan is a head-to-toe assessment and should include inspection, palpation, and auscultation as indicated.

➤ Remember to assess the posterior for any life-threatening conditions if not done during the primary assessment.

➤ Auscultate lung sounds, if not done earlier in the primary assessment.

vi. Transport priority

➤ Form your field impression, e.g., sick v. not sick.

➤ Do not delay transport of a high-priority patient to manage non-life-threatening conditions.

➤ A few significant MOIs indicating probable need for high-priority transport to an appropriate trauma center:

— Falls over 20 feet in adults or over 10 feet in children;

— Any fall leading to a traumatic loss of consciousness;

— Motor vehicle collisions (MVC) with more than 12″ of intrusion into occupant space;

— MVC with ejection;

— Death of another occupant in same vehicle;

— Pedestrian or cyclist struck by vehicle;

— Motorcycle accident over 20 mph.

> **Note:** Two or more significant MOIs significantly risk likelihood of life-threatening injury.

V. PATIENT HISTORY

A. For conscious medical patients, the most important information usually comes from the history.

B. Interpersonal communication

1. Do this:

    i. Introduce yourself and get patient's name (and use it).

    ii. Make eye contact.

    iii. Position yourself at same or lower level.

    iv. Be honest.

    v. Use appropriate language, terminology that the patient can understand.

    vi. Allow patient time to answer.

2. DON'T do this:

    i. Provide false assurance or lie.

    ii. Give advice.

    iii. Act authoritarian.

    iv. Use professional jargon.

    v. Use leading or biased questions.

    vi. Talk too much or interrupt.

    vii. Ask "why" questions.

C. **SAMPLE** history

1. Signs and symptoms

2. Allergies

3. Medications

4. Past history

5. Last oral intake

6. Events leading to incident

D. **OPQRST**

1. Onset

2. Provocation

3. Quality

4. Radiation

5. Severity

6. Time

E. ASPN

1. Associated symptoms: other symptoms associated with the chief complaint (e.g., chief complaint is chest pain, but patient also complains of dyspnea).

2. Pertinent negatives: potential associated symptoms that are not present (e.g., trauma patient denies neck pain).

 VI. **SECONDARY ASSESSMENT**

A. The four assessment techniques

1. Inspection: observation

2. Palpation: touch

3. Auscultation: listen

4. Percussion: not frequently used prehospital

B. Secondary assessment tips

1. The secondary assessment should not delay transport of a high priority patient.

2. The secondary assessment is designed to identify any remaining conditions or injuries.

3. The secondary assessment can be a detailed head-to-toe assessment or a focused assessment that assesses only relevant areas.

    i. Indications for a head-to-toe secondary assessment include:

        ➤ Unresponsive or otherwise unable to provide feedback

        ➤ Multisystem trauma

        ➤ High priority transport

    ii. Indications for a focused secondary assessment include conscious patients with a specific, isolated chief complaint (medical or trauma).

C. Body systems assessment

1. HEENT: head, eyes, ears, nose, throat

2. Chest and lungs

3. Abdomen (GI/GU)

4. Musculoskeletal

5. Neurological

6. Hematologic

7. Endocrine

8. Psychiatric

D. Assess for DCAP-BLS-TIC (trauma/unresponsive patients)

1. Inspect for:

    i. Deformities, distention

    ii. Contusion

    iii. Abrasion

iv. Penetrating injuries, paradoxical movement

v. Burns

vi. Laceration

vii. Swelling

2. Palpate for:

i. Tenderness

ii. Instability

iii. Crepitus

E. Baseline vitals

1. Respirations

2. Pulse

3. BP

4. Temperature

5. Skin

6. Pupils

7. Pulse oximetry, $ETCO_2$ (as indicated)

8. Blood glucose (as indicated)

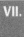 ## VII. REASSESSMENT

A. Reassessment tips

1. The purpose of the reassessment phase is to monitor for changes in the patient's condition.

2. Reassess stable patients every 15 minutes and unstable patients every 5 minutes.

3. Continue reassessment until transfer of care or until patient's condition requires repeat of the primary assessment.

B. Components of reassessment

1. Reassess LOC

2. Reassess ABCs

3. Reassess chief complaint

4. Reassess interventions

5. Reassess vitals

VIII. PRINCIPLES OF ALS MANAGEMENT

> **Note:** In later chapters, the information below will simply be referred to as "general management of ALS patients."

6. General management of ALS patients

   i. Manage ABCs as indicated

   ii. Supplemental oxygen and PPV as indicated

> **Note:** Always administer supplemental oxygen to patients with suspected hypoxia or shock. To avoid hyperoxia in stable patients, titrate oxygen to SpO_2 of 94%–99%.

   iii. Monitor ECG, SpO_2, $ETCO_2$ as indicated.

   iv. Assess blood glucose as indicated.

   v. IV access and fluid resuscitation (NaCl or LR) as indicated

   vi. Rapid transport as indicated

7. See appropriate chapters for specific interventions.

IX. PEDIATRIC ASSESSMENT TIPS

A. Infants (up to 1 year)

1. Should be alert and engaged with environment.

2. Arms and legs should move bilaterally.

3. Should recognize parents (over 2 months of age).

4. Normal vitals

   i. Respirations: 30–60

   ii. Heart rate: 100–180

   iii. Systolic BP: at least 70 to about 104

B. Toddlers (1–3 years)

1. Should be walking by 18 months.

2. Can often be disagreeable.

3. Most trusting of parents/guardians

4. May not want to be touched.

5. Focus on vital areas (based on complaint) first.

6. Normal vitals

   i.   Respirations: 24–40

   ii. Heart rate: 80–110

   iii. Systolic BP: about 80 + 2 (age in years)

C. Preschoolers (3–6 years)

1. Often distrust strangers.

2. May fear sight of blood, injury.

3. Answer questions honestly.

4. Normal vitals

   i.   Respirations: 22–34

   ii. Heart rate: 70–110

   iii. Systolic BP: about 80 + 2 (age in years)

D. School-age (6–12 years)

1. Often cooperative if they trust you.

2. Often seek control.

3. Offer choices.

4. May be modest, resist physical examination.

5. Normal vitals

   i.   Respirations: 18–30

   ii. Heart rate: 65–110

   iii. Systolic BP: about 80 + 2 (age in years)

E. Adolescent (13–18 years)

    1. Treat similar to adults.

    2. Can be extremely modest.

    3. Consider same-sex provider if possible.

    4. Normal vitals

        i.   Respirations: 12–26

        ii. Heart rate: 60–90

        iii. Systolic BP: 110–130

X. SUMMARY OF PATIENT ASSESSMENT

A. Scene size-up

    1. Scene safety, standard precautions

    2. Number of patients, additional resources

    3. Consider MOI or NOI

B. Primary assessment

    1. ABCs or CAB (if unresponsive)

    2. Rapid scan as indicated

    3. Determine transport priority.

C. Patient history (may come before or after secondary assessment)

    1. SAMPLE

D. Secondary assessment

    1. Detailed assessment or focused assessment (as indicated)

E. Reassessment

    1. Reassess patient's chief complaint, vitals, interventions, etc.

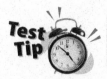

Be sure to know the "general management of ALS (Advanced Life Support) patients" referred to throughout the book. These are the foundational assessments and interventions for paramedics.

Patient Monitoring Technology

I. TERMS TO KNOW

A. Capnography—measure or monitoring of exhaled CO_2

B. Infarct—area of necrosis, or death

C. Pulse CO-oximetry (SpCO)—non-invasive measurement of carbon monoxide saturation of hemoglobin

D. Pulse oximetry (SpO_2)—non-invasive measurement of oxygen saturation of hemoglobin

E. SpMet—non-invasive measurement of methemoglobin

II. PATIENT MONITORING TECHNIQUES USED IN PREHOSPITAL

A. ECG monitoring and 12-lead ECG

B. Pulse oximetry

C. Pulse CO-oximetry

D. Capnography

E. Methemoglobin monitoring

F. Total hemoglobin monitoring

G. Glucometry

III. ECG MONITORING

A. Bipolar leads

1. Lead I: negative electrode right arm and positive electrode left arm

2. Lead II: negative electrode right arm and positive electrode left leg

3. Lead III: negative electrode left arm and positive electrode left leg

B. Limitations

1. Provides no information regarding mechanical cardiac function.

2. Non-diagnostic for MI

IV. 12-LEAD ECG

A. Advantages

1. Diagnostic for myocardial ischemia, injury, infarct

2. Can provide earlier recognition and management of ST-segment elevation myocardial infarction (STEMI).

3. Can flag a possible cardiac problem.

> *Note:* ECG changes must occur in at least two contiguous leads (see lead groupings).

B. Limitations

1. Provides no information regarding mechanical cardiac function.

2. Standard 12-lead provides limited information about right ventricle and posterior left ventricle.

C. Zones of myocardial damage

1. Ischemia

    i.   Myocardium receiving inadequate oxygen (reversible condition)

    ii. ECG: ST depression, inverted T waves or peaked T waves

> *Note:* ST depression must be at least one small box below baseline.

2. Injury

    i.   Myocardial damage due to ischemia (potentially reversible condition)

    ii. ECG: ST elevation.

> *Note:* ST elevation must be at least 1 mm in two or more continuous leads or inverted T waves.

3. Infarction

    i.   Myocardial death (irreversible condition)

    ii. ECG: significant (pathological) Q wave

> *Note:* Pathological Q wave must be at least 1 mm (0.04 seconds) wide or deeper than one-third the R wave (in same lead).

D. Lead placement (12-lead)

1. Bipolar leads—I, II, III

2. Unipolar (augmented) leads—aVR, aVL, aVF

3. Chest (precordial) leads—V$_1$–V$_6$

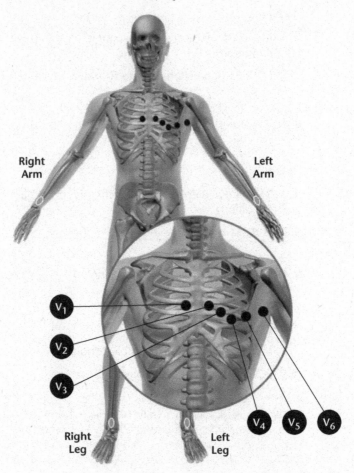

Electrode	Placement Area
V$_1$	Fourth intercostal space to the right of the sternum.
V$_2$	Fourth intercostal space to the left of the sternum.
V$_3$	Directly between leads V$_2$ and V$_4$.
V$_4$	Fifth intercostal space at midclavicular line.
V$_5$	Level with V$_4$ at left anterior axillary line.
V$_6$	Level with V$_5$ at the midaxillary line. (Directly under the midpoint of the armpit)

4. Lead groupings ("I See All Leads" mnemonic)

    i.   Inferior leads: leads II, III, aVF

    ii. Septal leads: V_1, V_2

    iii. Anterior leads: V_3, V_4

    iv. Lateral leads: lead I, aVL, V_5, V_6

V. PULSE OXIMETRY (SPO₂)

A. Uses

1. Non-invasive and indirect method of monitoring oxygen saturation of hemoglobin (SpO_2)

    i. SpO_2 readings are a percentage, therefore max value is 100.

    ii. SaO_2 (unlike SpO_2) is a direct and invasive measurement (arterial blood gas). (Easy to confuse these, but medics use SpO_2.)

2. Monitoring of pulse rate

    i.   Unlike an ECG, the SpO_2 monitor *can* provide info about mechanical cardiac function.

    ii. Most SpO_2 devices provide visual and auditory monitoring of pulse (that annoying, but sometimes helpful "BEEP"). Example: auditory monitoring of pulse for possible bradycardia in pediatric patients or newborns.

3. SpO_2 could be useful in assessing circulation distal to a suspected orthopedic fracture or for identifying inapparent hypoxia in patients with long bone fractures.

B. SpO_2 values

1. Normal—95%–100%

2. Below 95%—suspect hypoxia, shock, or respiratory compromise

3. Below 90%—aggressive airway management, ventilatory support and high-flow oxygen indicated

> **Note:** COPD patients may routinely have SpO_2 readings as low as 85%.

4. Indications

    i. Dyspnea or other indications of respiratory compromise

    ii. Suspected hypoxia

    iii. ALOC

    iv. Suspected shock, multi-system trauma

    v. Traumatic brain injury

    vi. Suspected MI or stroke

    vii. Patients receiving analgesics or sedation medications

    viii. Any patient receiving supplemental oxygen or PPV

    ix. Possible identification of inapparent hypoxia after long bone fractures

    x. Use to maintain patient's SpO_2 at 95% or above

> **Note:** Excessive oxygen administration can have harmful effects (vasoconstriction, free radicals). Consider titrating to 95% instead of 100% to reduce risk of complications.

5. Limitations

    i. Inaccurate readings possible due to

        ➤ Hypoperfusion (Example: hemorrhage, dehydration, hypothermia)

        ➤ Anemia (An SpO_2 of 100% in a patient without enough RBCs is *not* good.)

        ➤ CO poisoning (Device only reads percentage on bound hemoglobin, not what is bound to that hemoglobin, e.g., O_2 v. CO.)

        ➤ Methemoglobinemia/cyanide poisoning

    ii. Does not indicate total respiratory or circulatory sufficiency, must be used with other assessments, physical exam, etc.

    iii. There can be a delay in desaturation readings (not an immediate, real-time indicator of patient's condition).

VI. CAPNOGRAPHY

A. $ETCO_2$ provides real-time information regarding cellular metabolism, circulation, and ventilation.

> **Note:** Capnography and capnometry are often used synonymously; however, capnography indicates continuous monitoring (numerical or waveform), while capnometry indicates analysis without continuous monitoring.

B. $ETCO_2$ values

1. Normal $ETCO_2$ — 35–45 mmHg
2. Elevated $ETCO_2$ (greater than 45 mmHg)
   i. Elevated $ETCO_2$ indicates hypoventilation due to:
      ➤ increased CO_2 production and/or
      ➤ decreased CO_2 elimination
   ii. Elevated $ETCO_2$ indicates acidosis
3. Decreased $ETCO_2$ (below 35 mmHg)
   i. Decreased $ETCO_2$ indicates hyperventilation due to:
      ➤ decreased CO_2 production and/or
      ➤ increased CO_2 elimination
   ii. Decreased $ETCO_2$ indicates alkalosis

C. Capnography devices

1. Colorimetric devices
   i. Disposable, color-changing $ETCO_2$ detector
   ii. Used to help verify ETT placement or indicate displacement of ETT.
   iii. Limitations are extensive, such as no numerical value and no waveform.
2. Electronic capnography can provide a numerical value or a numerical value and a waveform.

D. Indications and advantages of continuous $ETCO_2$ monitoring

1. Continuously monitor ETT

2. Monitor effectiveness of CPR

3. Monitor adequacy of ventilations

4. Improved management of patients with increased ICP, especially if patient is being ventilated (adjust ventilations to target $ETCO_2$ of 40 mmHg).

VII. PULSE CO-OXIMETRY (SPCO)

A. Carbon monoxide (CO) binds to hemoglobin much stronger (200x) than oxygen does, causing carboxyhemoglobin (a common toxicologic emergency).

B. Firefighters at increased risk of chronic and acute exposure to CO.

C. Pulse CO-oximetry (SpCO) provides rapid, noninvasive detection of CO poisoning

1. SpCO devices also provide SpO_2 and pulse rate data.

D. SpCO values and interventions

1. 0%–3%—normal

2. 3%–12%—Administer high-flow oxygen and transport if symptomatic, or known exposure to CO.

3. Above 12%—Administer high-flow oxygen and transport.

> **Notes:**
>
> —Any symptomatic patient with known CO exposure should be transported, regardless of SpCO reading.
>
> —At least mild symptoms are present once carboxyhemoglobin (COHb) reaches about 15%.
>
> —Consider hyperbaric chamber for patients with excessively high SpCO, especially pediatric patients and pregnant females.

E. Indications

1. Known or suspected exposure to CO

2. Persistent hypoxia despite oxygen therapy

3. Altered LOC of unknown etiology

F. Limitations: similar to SpO_2 devices

 VIII. **METHEMOGLOBINEMIA (SPMET) MONITORING**

A. High levels of methemoglobin (MetHb) disrupt the hemoglobin's ability to transport and deliver oxygen to the cells, causing hypoxia.

B. Some SpCO monitors can measure MetHb levels (measured as SpMet).

C. SpMet values

1. 1%–3% SpMet—normal

2. 3%–15% SpMet—ashen or cyanotic skin possible

3. 15%–20% SpMet—cyanosis

4. 25%–50% SpMet—headache, dyspnea, ALOC

5. 50%–70% SpMet—Altered or decreased LOC

6. 70% or above—Fatal

D. Indications

1. Cyanosis unresolved by oxygen therapy

2. Patients receiving IV nitrates, lidocaine, nitric oxide (NO)

3. Suspected cyanide exposure

4. Any patient with elevated SpCO levels

E. Limitations: similar to SpO_2 and SpCO devices

1. Elevated SpMet levels in the blood can result in a falsely elevated SpCO reading.

IX. TOTAL HEMOGLOBIN MONITORING

A. Some SpCO monitors can measure total hemoglobin concentrations (measured as SpHb) and help identify patients with dehydration or hemorrhage.

B. Normal hemoglobin (Hb) values are age-dependent

1. Newborns–2 weeks: 14.5–24.5 g/dL

2. Infants up to 8 weeks: 12.5–20.5 g/dL

3. Infants up to 6 months: 10.7–17.3 g/dL

4. Infants up to 1 year: 9.9–14.5 g/dL

5. Children up to 6 years: 9.5–14.1 g/dL

6. Adult males: 14–17.4 g/dL

7. Adult females: 12–16 g/dL

C. Abnormal SpHb (Remember, SpHb is the indirect, noninvasive measure of Hb levels.)

1. High SpHb—suspect dehydration (hemoconcentration due to low plasma)

2. Low SpHb—suspect hemorrhage, anemia

D. Indications for SpHb monitoring

1. Suspected dehydration or hemorrhage

2. Suspected hypoperfusion (shock)

X. GLUCOMETRY

A. Indications

1. Known or suspected diabetic history

2. Altered or decreased LOC

3. Seizures

4. Stroke

5. Pregnancy

      6. Suspected alcohol abuse

      7. Suspected overdose

      8. Any time you have any reason to remotely suspect an abnormal blood glucose level (It's fast, easy, and minimally invasive.)

B. Blood glucose values

      1. Normal (adult, non-diabetic)—about 70–120 mg/dL

      2. Normal (adult, diabetic)—about 100–180 mg/dL

      3. Normal (newborn)—above 40 mg/dL

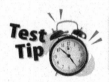

The certification exam places a strong emphasis on anatomy, physiology, pathophysiology, and terminology. Be sure to review the "Terms to Know" at the beginning of each chapter and "Anatomy and Physiology Review" sections in this book.

Bleeding and Shock

> *Note:* For information about general management of ALS patients, see Chapter 4.

I. TERMS TO KNOW

A. Angioedema—swelling of the lower layer of skin and underlying tissue. Swelling may occur in the face, tongue, larynx, abdomen, arms and legs. Often associated with urticaria.

B. Compensated shock—early shock where the body still maintains adequate perfusion

C. Decompensated shock—later shock where the body can no longer maintain adequate perfusion

D. Exsanguination—severe bleeding, leading to death

E. Hemorrhage—bleeding

F. Irreversible shock—stage of shock leading to inevitable death

G. Mean arterial pressure (MAP)—DBP + 1/3 (SBP − DBP)

H. Multiple organ dysfunction syndrome—progressive failure of at least two organ systems

I. Urticaria—hives

II. BLEEDING

A. Types of bleeding

1. External

   i.   Check for bleeding from places that may not be obvious, e.g., posterior, axillary regions.

   > *Note:* Remember to expose any patient with suspected bleeding.

2. Internal

   i.   A single femur fracture, pelvic fracture, or multiple long bone fractures can lead to hemorrhagic shock.

   ii. Signs of internal hemorrhage

   - ➤ Vomiting blood
   - ➤ Coffee ground-like emesis
   - ➤ Blood in stool (hematochezia)
   - ➤ Dark, tarry stool (melena)
   - ➤ Abdominal distention or rigidity
   - ➤ Suspected femur or pelvic fracture
   - ➤ Signs and symptoms of shock

B. Sources of bleeding

1. Arterial bleeding—spurting, bright red blood

2. Venous bleeding—steady flowing, dark red

3. Capillary bleeding—slow, oozing dark red blood

C. Management of bleeding

1. External bleeding

   i.   First method: direct pressure

   - ➤ Consider hemostatic dressings and/or wound packing per local protocol.

ii.   Second method: tourniquet

➤ Use commercial tourniquet if available and per local protocol.

➤ Can use BP cuff as last resort (monitor for leaks).

➤ Always place tourniquet proximal to injury.

➤ Apply enough pressure to control bleeding.

➤ Do not apply directly over joint.

➤ Write "TK" and time applied on tape and secure to patient's forehead and notify transfer of care personnel.

2.   Suspected internal bleeding

i.   General management of ALS patients

ii.   Treat for shock

iii.   Consider pelvic binder for suspected pelvic fracture

iv.   Rapid transport

III.   SHOCK

A. Shock (aka hypoperfusion) is any condition causing inadequate tissue perfusion due to reduced cardiac output.

B. Three primary causes of shock (aka the "Perfusion Triangle")

1. Pump (cardiac) problem (e.g., cardiogenic shock)

2. Pipes (vasodilation) problem (e.g., anaphylactic shock)

3. Fluid (hypovolemic) problem (e.g., hemorrhagic shock)

C. Impaired Oxygenation and Glucose

1. All causes of shock lead to impaired oxygenation due to anaerobic (without oxygen) metabolic function.

2. Anaerobic metabolism creates little energy and increased acidosis.

3. Shock also causes impaired glucose delivery to cells, increasing risk of organ failure.

IV. CATEGORIES (STAGES) OF SHOCK

A. Compensated shock

1. The body's defense mechanisms are compensating for the decrease in cardiac output.

2. Compensatory mechanisms

   i. Increased heart rate and cardiac force of contraction

   ii. Increased vasoconstriction

   iii. Reduced urinary output to maintain intravascular volume

B. Decompensated (progressive) shock

1. The body's defense mechanisms are no longer able to compensate for the decrease in cardiac output.

2. Falling or low BP are hallmark signs of decompensated shock.

3. Importance of mean arterial pressure (MAP)

   i. $MAP = DBP + \frac{1}{3}(SBP - DBP)$

   ii. Normal MAP is 70–100. A MAP of at least 60 is needed to perfuse vital organs.

C. Irreversible Shock

1. Irrecoverable shock leading to inevitable death

V. CLASSIFICATION (TYPES) OF SHOCK

A. Older classification system

1. Cardiogenic shock (pump problem)

2. Hypovolemic shock (fluid problem)

3. Neurogenic shock (vasodilation problem)

4. Anaphylactic shock (vasodilation/permeability problem)

5. Septic shock (vasodilation/permeability problem)

B. Newer classification system

1. Cardiogenic shock

2. Hypovolemic shock

3. Obstructive shock

   i.   Pulmonary embolism

   ii. Cardiac tamponade

   iii. Tension pneumothorax

4. Distributive shock

   i.   Neurogenic shock

   ii. Anaphylactic shock

   iii. Septic shock

VI. SIGNS, SYMPTOMS AND MANAGEMENT OF SHOCK

A. Classic signs of shock

1. Altered LOC progressing to unresponsiveness

2. Tachycardia progressing to absent pulses in decompensated/irreversible shock

3. Pale, cool, clammy skin

4. Normal BP during compensated shock and falling BP during decompensated shock

5. Differentiating Compensated v. Decompensated Shock

   i.   Signs and symptoms of compensated shock

      ➤ Altered LOC (restless, anxious, irritable)

      ➤ Tachycardia

      ➤ Pale, cool, clammy skin

      ➤ Thirst

      ➤ *Normal* blood pressure

   ii. Signs and symptoms of decompensated shock

      ➤ Decreased LOC

      ➤ Absent peripheral pulses

      ➤ Mottling, cyanosis

      ➤ *Falling* blood pressure progressing to *hypotension*

B. Standard Shock Management

1. Airway management, supplemental oxygen, ventilation support as indicated

2. Control bleeding as indicated.

3. Prevent heat loss (even mild hypothermia increases metabolic demand and inhibits clotting).

4. Rapid transport

5. IV access

6. Consider IV fluid bolus using volume expanders (such as normal saline or lactated Ringers).

   i. Rule out pulmonary edema before IV fluid challenge.

   ii. Fluid bolus not typically indicated for adults with SBP of at least 100 mmHg

   iii. If indicated (SBP 90 or below for adults), consider 250 mL fluid bolus.

   iv. Burn patients—see Burn chapter

   v. Pediatric patients—see Pediatrics chapter

C. Cardiogenic Shock

1. Left ventricular failure is the most common cause.

2. Signs and symptoms

   i. Classic signs of shock

   ii. Dyspnea and pulmonary edema

   iii. Cyanosis

3. Management

   i. Standard shock management

D. Hypovolemic Shock

1. Causes include hemorrhage, vomiting, diarrhea, burns, sweating, DKA

2. Signs and symptoms

   i. Classic signs of shock

3. Management

   i.   Classic management

   ii. IV fluids

      ➤ IV fluids indicated for most causes of hypovolemic shock with presenting hypotension; however, specific guidelines vary and are still controversial (search "permissive hypotension" for additional info).

      ➤ Permissive hypotension

         — Research on permissive hypotension is currently inconclusive. However, there are indications of possible improved outcomes for patients whose BP is maintained at not greater than about 90 systolic.

         — Follow local protocols regarding IV fluid resuscitation for shock and trauma patients.

      ➤ Pediatric fluid resuscitation

         — Infants—10 mL/kg

         — Pediatrics—20 mL/kg

E. Neurogenic Shock

1. Damage to brain or spinal cord leading to widespread vasodilation and relative hypovolemia

2. Signs and symptoms

   i.   Possible paralysis

   ii. Possible respiratory compromise

   iii. MOI indicative of probable spinal injury

   iv. Warm, flushed, dry skin (*not* pale, cool, clammy skin as usually seen)

   v. Hypotension even in early stage of shock

   vi. Slow pulse (*not* the tachycardia usually seen)

Note: The three unique characteristics of neurogenic shock are early hypotension, bradycardia, and warm, dry skin.

3. Management

    i.   Standard shock management

F. Anaphylactic Shock

    1.   Life-threatening allergic reaction to an antigen, such as food, meds, venom

    2.   Signs and symptoms

        i.   Skin: flushed, itching, urticaria, angioedema

        ii.   Respiratory: dyspnea, wheezing, stridor, laryngospasm

        iii. Cardiovascular: widespread vasodilation, tachycardia

    3.   Management

        i.   Aggressive airway intervention likely needed due to laryngospasm

        ii.   High-flow oxygen and ventilatory support as indicated

        iii. Epinephrine

        iv. IV fluids for volume support

        v.   Consider antihistamines, steroids per local protocol

Note: The three acute life-threats caused by anaphylaxis are airway compromise (laryngospasm); respiratory compromise (bronchoconstriction/edema); and circulatory compromise (massive vasodilation).

G. Septic Shock (Sepsis)

    1.   Systemic infection that enters the blood and is carried throughout the body

    2.   Signs and symptoms

        i.   Fever or hypothermia possible

        ii.   Skin can be flushed, pale, or cyanotic.

        iii. ALOC

        iv. Dyspnea, abnormal lung sounds

        v.   Tachycardia, hypotension

3. Management

    i.   Standard shock management and IV fluid support

Shock Cycle

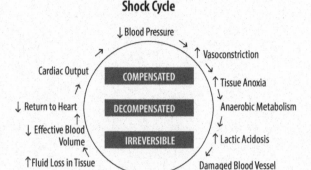

VII. MULTIPLE ORGAN DYSFUNCTION SYNDROME

A. Multiple organ failure following conditions such as shock, trauma, burns, surgery, renal failure

B. Major cause of death following sepsis, significant trauma, and major burns

C. Early stages present with fever, ALOC, tachycardia, dyspnea.

D. Later stages present with systems failure, moving from pulmonary to hepatic, intestinal, renal and finally cardiac failure, encephalopathy, and death.

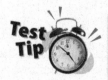

Security on the National Certification exam is rigorous. The questions come from an extensive unpublished database. There is no way to view these questions in advance. The keys to passing the exam are possession of the necessary knowledge and good test-taking skills. This book will help with both!

PART III

MEDICAL EMERGENCIES
UNIT 1

Cardiology and Resuscitation

Note: For information about general management of ALS patients, see Chapter 4.

I. CARDIOLOGY

A. Terms to Know

1. Afterload—resistance the left heart overcomes during contraction

2. Aneurysm—a weakening in the wall of an artery

3. Ascites—edema in the abdomen

4. Cardiac hypertrophy—enlargement of the heart, often due to hypertension

5. Cardiac output—volume of blood ejected by left ventricle in one minute (stroke volume x heart rate)

6. Chronotrope—rate of cardiac contraction

7. Dromotrope—speed of cardiac conduction velocity

8. Endocarditis—an infection of the endocardium, usually involving the heart valves

9. Ejection fraction—percentage of blood ejected from a filled ventricle

10. Failure to capture—ventricles fail to respond to an impulse. On an ECG, the pacemaker spike will appear, but it will not be followed by a QRS complex

11. Failure to sense—pacemaker malfunction that occurs when the pacemaker does not detect the patient's myocardial depolarization. May be seen on an ECG tracing as a spike following a QRS complex too early

12. Inotrope—force of cardiac contraction

13. Orthopnea—difficulty breathing while supine

14. Paroxysmal nocturnal dyspnea—acute onset of difficulty breathing at night, usually while sleeping

15. Pericarditis—Inflammation of the pericardium

16. Preload—volume of fluid returning to the right heart

17. Prinzmetal's angina—variable angina caused by coronary artery spasms

18. Starling's law—the more the heart is stretched (within limits), the greater the resulting force of contraction

19. Stroke volume—amount of blood ejected by left ventricle during one contraction

B. Risk Factors for Heart Disease

1. Smoking

2. Hypertension

3. Age (risk increases with age)

4. High cholesterol

5. Diabetes

6. Heredity

7. Gender (increased risk for males)

8. Substance abuse

9. Lack of exercise

10. Oral contraceptives

11. Stress

C. Anatomy and Physiology Review

1. Layers of the heart

    i. Endocardium—innermost layer

ii. Myocardium—muscular wall of the heart

iii. Epicardium—inner layer of the pericardial sac

iv. Pericardium—outer layer of the pericardial sac

2. Blood flow through the heart

   i. Oxygen-rich blood exits the left side of the heart through the aorta.

   ii. The aorta branches off into arteries, then arterioles, and finally capillaries. On the venous side, capillaries feed into venules, then veins, and finally the superior or inferior vena cava.

The Pathway of Blood Flow Through the Heart

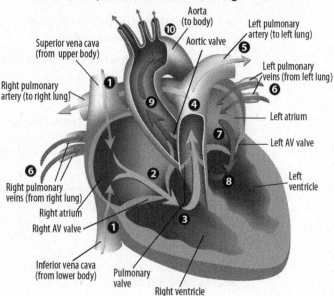

Figure 7.1

iii. Figure 7.1 shows the pathway of blood flow through the heart. The vena cava (1) returns blood to the right side of the heart into the right atrium (2). The right atrium pumps blood into the right ventricle (3), which pumps deoxygenated blood through the pulmonary arteries (4) and (5) into the lungs. The carbon dioxide and oxygen exchange takes place between the alveoli and the pulmonary capillaries. Oxygen-rich blood from the lungs returns to the left chamber of the heart through the pulmonary veins (6) into the left atrium (7). The left atrium pumps blood into the left ventricle (8), which then pumps it to the aorta (9) and (10) for circulation throughout the body.

iv. Arteries always carry blood away from the heart, and veins always carry blood toward the heart. Note that the pulmonary artery is the one artery in the body that carries deoxygenated blood. The pulmonary vein is the only vein in the body that carries oxygen-rich blood.

3. Systemic vascular resistance (SVR)

i. SVR is the resistance to blood flow throughout the body (excluding the pulmonary system).

ii. SVR is determined by the size of blood vessels.

➤ Constriction of blood vessels increases SVR and can cause an increase in blood pressure.

➤ Dilation of blood vessels decreases SVR and can lower blood pressure.

4. Preload and afterload

i. Preload: the pre-contraction pressure based on the volume of blood coming back to the heart. Increased preload increases stretching of the ventricles and increased myocardial contractility.

ii. Afterload: the resistance the heart must overcome during ventricular contraction. Increased afterload decreases cardiac output.

5. Coronary circulation

i. The heart receives its own blood supply through the coronary arteries during diastole.

ii. Left coronary artery (LCA): typically, the LCA perfuses left ventricle, interventricular septum, portion of the right ventricle, and the cardiac conduction system. Main branches of the LCA are the left anterior descending (LAD) artery and the left circumflex artery.

iii. Right coronary artery (RCA): typically, the RCA perfuses part of right atrium and ventricle, and part of cardiac conduction system. Main branches of RCA are the posterior descending artery and the right marginal artery.

6. Cardiac conduction

   i. Sinoatrial (SA) node: the heart's primary conduction system. Typically generates electrical impulses between 60–100 times per minute.

   ii. Atrioventricular (AV) junction: the heart's first backup pacemaker. Typically generates electrical impulses between 40–60 times per minute.

   iii. Bundle of His: the heart's final pacemaker. Typically generates electrical impulses at 20–40 per minute.

   iv. ECG Interpretation

1. Basic ECG interpretation cannot be adequately covered in this review text; however, here are the rhythm categories and dysrhythmias you should be familiar with:

   i. Sinus rhythms and dysrhythmias

       ➤ Sinus rhythm

       ➤ Sinus bradycardia

       ➤ Sinus tachycardia

       ➤ Sinus block

       ➤ Sinus arrest

   ii. Atrial rhythms and dysrhythmias

       ➤ Supraventricular tachycardia

       ➤ Paroxysmal supraventricular tachycardia (intermittent)

       ➤ Atrial flutter

       ➤ Atrial fibrillation

       ➤ Premature atrial contractions

       ➤ Wandering atrial pacemaker

       ➤ Multifocal atrial tachycardia

   iii. AV blocks

       ➤ 1st degree AV block

       ➤ 2nd degree AV block type I

       ➤ 2nd degree AV block type II

       ➤ 2nd degree AV block 2:1 conduction

       ➤ 3rd degree AV block

    iv. Junctional rhythms and dysrhythmias

- Junctional escape rhythm
- Junctional bradycardia
- Accelerated junctional rhythm
- Premature junctional complexes
- Junctional escape complexes
- Junctional escape rhythm

    v. Ventricular rhythms and dysrhythmias

- Accelerated idioventricular rhythm
- Ventricular tachycardia
- Ventricular fibrillation
- Torsades de pointes
- Ventricular escape complexes
- Ventricular escape rhythm
- Premature ventricular complexes

    vi. Additional rhythms and dysrhythmias

- Asystole
- Artificial pacemaker rhythms

  2. 12-lead ECG: see Chapter 5: Patient Monitoring Technology.

E. Common Signs and Symptoms of Cardiac Emergencies

1. Chest pain or pressure
2. Dyspnea
3. Palpitations
4. Diaphoresis
5. Restlessness, anxiety
6. Feeling of impending doom
7. Nausea and vomiting
8. Weakness

9. Edema

10. Syncope

11. Denial

F. General management of cardiac emergencies

   1. Assess and manage ABCs.

   2. BLS and ACLS interventions as indicated for cardiac arrest

   3. Supplemental oxygen as indicated to maintain SpO_2 of at least 95%

   4. Continuous ECG monitoring/serial 12-lead ECG

   5. IV access and pharmacological interventions as indicated (e.g., aspirin, nitroglycerine)

   6. Rapid transport to the closest appropriate facility

G. Management of cardiac dysrhythmias

   1. Determine if patient is symptomatic, e.g., altered LOC, hypotensive, chest pain, etc.

   2. Follow appropriate ACLS algorithm.

      i.   Consider vagal maneuvers for tachydysrhythmias.

      ii. Consider appropriate pharmacological interventions.

      iii. Consider appropriate electrical interventions, e.g., cardioversion, defibrillation, transcutaneous external pacing.

H. Acute Coronary Syndrome (ACS)

   1. ACS includes angina, unstable angina, and acute myocardial infarction.

   2. Angina (stable angina)

      i.   Transient chest pain due to myocardial ischemia

      ii. Often provoked by exertion or stress

      iii. Typically lasts less than 30 minutes and resolved with rest or nitroglycerine

   3. Unstable angina

      i.   presents with at least *one* of the following

           ➤ New onset angina

➤ Angina for at least 20 minutes while at rest

➤ Frequent angina episodes or increasing duration of angina

4. Acute myocardial infarction (AMI)

   i. AMI is irreversible necrosis of myocardial muscle and diagnosed by ECG changes and elevated myocardial blood enzymes.

   ii. AMI classification is based on ECG findings

➤ ST elevation MI (STEMI)

➤ Non-ST elevation MI (NSTEMI)

   iii. Use caution when considering nitroglycerine in suspected right ventricular inferior MI (risk of profound hypotension). Follow local protocol.

I. Congestive heart failure (CHF)

1. Left heart failure

   i. Left ventricular dysfunction causes backpressure into pulmonary circulation.

   ii. Dyspnea and pulmonary edema are common with left heart failure.

   iii. Myocardial infarction is a common cause of left heart failure.

2. Right heart failure

   i. Right ventricular dysfunction causes backpressure into systemic venous circulation.

   ii. JVD and pedal edema are common with right heart failure.

   iii. Left heart failure is the most frequent cause of right heart failure.

3. Signs and symptoms of CHF

   i. Pulmonary edema (typically left heart failure)

   ii. Dyspnea (typically left heart failure)

   iii. Paroxysmal nocturnal dyspnea (typically left heart failure)

   iv. Orthopnea (typically left heart failure)

   v. Mottled skin

   vi. Weakness

   vii. Ascites (typically right heart failure)

viii. JVD (typically right heart failure)

ix. Bilateral pedal edema (typically right heart failure)

x. Patients with a history of CHF are often prescribed medications such as digoxin (positive inotrope), a diuretic (such as furosemide), an ACE inhibitor, and a potassium supplement.

> *Note:* Be very clear on the signs and symptoms that distinguish left vs. right heart failure and remember, some patients can have bilateral heart failure.

4. Management of CHF

Left Heart Failure	Right Heart Failure
• Dyspnea	• JVD
• Pulmonary edema	• Pedal edema

i. Avoid placing patient supine.

ii. Supplemental oxygen as indicated.

iii. Continuous positive airway pressure (CPAP) as indicated starting with 5 cm H_2O and up to 10 cm H_2O if needed.

iv. ECG monitoring

v. IV access

vi. Nitroglycerine as indicated.

vii. Use of narcotics and diuretics in CHF patients has been shown to be ineffective and possibly harmful.

J. Cardiac Tamponade

1. Excess fluid accumulation in the pericardial sac impairing diastolic filling and reducing cardiac output.

2. Causes can be medical or trauma related.

3. Signs and symptoms

i. Chest pain

ii. Dyspnea

iii. Beck's triad: JVD, narrowing pulse pressure, muffled heart tones

> **Note:** For any patient with JVD and clear lung sounds, be alert for possible right ventricular infarct, pulmonary embolism, or cardiac tamponade.

4. Management

    i. High-flow oxygen

    ii. IV fluids if hypotensive

    iii. Consider vasopressors, such as dopamine.

    iv. Rapid transport

K. Hypertensive Emergencies

1. Signs and symptoms

    i. Elevation in blood pressure (>180/120) with some sort of target organ change, such as:

- ALOC
- Headache
- Dyspnea
- Chest pain
- Vomiting
- Visual disturbance
- Pulmonary edema
- ECG changes
- Symptoms of stroke
- Seizures

    ii. History of hypertensive disorder

    iii. Noncompliance with anti-hypertensive meds

    iv. Pregnancy (preeclampsia and pregnancy induced hypertension)

    v. Nosebleed

2. Management

    i.   Manage airway, breathing, circulation as indicated.

    ii.   Supplemental oxygen as indicated.

    iii.   Place in position of comfort (pregnant patients left lateral recumbent).

    iv.   IV access (do not delay transport to establish IV)

    v.   Transport.

L. Abdominal Aortic Aneurysm (AAA)

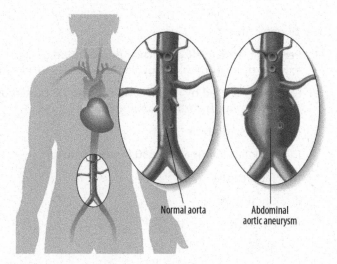

Normal aorta   Abdominal aortic aneurysm

1. Aortic aneurysms often occur in the abdominal region, but can also develop along the thoracic aorta (thoracic aortic aneurysm), or in the brain (cerebral aneurysm).

2. The weakened wall of the affected artery is prone to rupture and massive bleeding.

3. Signs and symptoms of AAA

    i.   Most common in older males

    ii.   Tearing back pain

    iii.   Possible history of hypertension, smoking, atherosclerosis, family history of AAA

    iv.   Possible pulsating abdominal mass

      v.   Varying blood pressures between left and right arm of (at least 15–20 mmHg)

      vi. Signs and symptoms of hypovolemic shock (if ruptured)

  4. Management

      i.   General management of ALS patients

      ii.   Keep patient still.

      iii. Caution when palpating abdomen

      iv. Transport rapidly to appropriate facility with surgical capabilities.

M. Cardiogenic Shock

  1. Persistent, severe left ventricular pump failure despite correction of existing dysrhythmias, hypovolemia, or widespread vasodilation

  2. Frequently caused by massive MI; can also be caused by tension pneumothorax or cardiac tamponade

  3. Signs and symptoms

      i.   Hypotension (may be <80 mmHg systolic)

      ii.   Tachycardia

      iii. Chest pain

      iv. Dyspnea

      v.   ALOC

      vi. Weakness

      vii. History of trauma or MI

  4. Management

      i.   Manage airway, breathing, circulation as indicated.

      ii.   Position of comfort if possible

      iii. Oxygen as indicated

      iv. Consider CPAP.

      v.   Consider vasopressor medication, such as dopamine.

      vi. Rapid transport to appropriate facility

II. RESUSCITATION

A. The national certification exam is based on the current American Heart Association guidelines for Basic Life Support, Emergency Cardiovascular Care, and Advanced Cardiac Life Support.

B. Highlights of current AHA BLS guidelines

1. Rate of chest compression—100–120 per minute (adults and peds)

2. Depth of compression adults—2–2.4" (5–6 cm)

3. Depth of compression children—2" (5 cm)

4. Depth of compression infants—1.5" (4 cm)

5. Adult compression to ventilation ratio—30:2 (one or two rescuers)

6. Infant and child comp:vent ratio—30:2 (one rescuer); 15:2 (two rescuers)

7. Ventilation rate with advanced airway—10/minute (adults); 12–20/minute (peds)

8. Ensure full chest recoil between compressions.

9. Minimize interruptions in chest compressions (10 seconds or less).

10. Avoid hyperventilation.

11. Utilize AED to determine need for defibrillation as early as possible.

12. Oxygen should be administered to maintain SpO_2 of at least 94% (but less than 100% after return of spontaneous circulation (ROSC)).

13. Evidence does not demonstrate benefit of mechanical CPR devices over manual CPR.

14. Routine suctioning of newborns not indicated.

C. Highlights of current AHA ACLS guidelines

1. Vasopressin no longer recommended for cardiac arrest.

2. Amiodarone or lidocaine may be used for VF or pulseless VT after CPR, defibrillation, and epinephrine.

3. Consider termination of efforts if unable to obtain $ETCO_2$ above 10 mmHg in an intubated patient after 20 minutes of CPR.

4. Atropine indicated for symptomatic bradycardia (ALOC, chest pain, hypotension)

5. Consider dopamine or epinephrine infusion or transcutaneous external pacing (TEP) for symptomatic bradycardia unresponsive to atropine.

6. Consider immediate TEP for symptomatic bradycardia with high-degree AV block when IV access delayed.

7. 12-lead ECG should be obtained prehospital for suspected acute coronary syndrome to assess for STEMI.

D. Highlights of current AHA PALS guidelines

1. Early, rapid administration of isotonic IV fluids at 20 mL/kg recommended for pediatric patients with hypovolemia or sepsis

2. Amiodarone or lidocaine can be used for shock-refractory VT or pulseless VT.

3. Administer oxygen as indicated to maintain SpO_2 between 94%–99%.

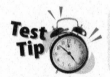

Test Tip

Go to NREMT.org. Search for a page titled "NREMT implements AHA guidelines." This is a gold mine of flashcard material related to BLS, ACLS, and PALS content you can expect to see on the certification exam.

Pulmonology

I

TERMS TO KNOW

A. Acute respiratory distress syndrome (ARDS)—non-cardiogenic pulmonary edema

B. Cor pulmonale—right-heart failure

C. Hemoptysis—coughing up blood

D. Orthopnea—difficulty breathing while lying down

E. Paroxysmal nocturnal dyspnea—difficulty breathing at night

F. Positive end-expiratory pressure (PEEP)—Extrinsic PEEP uses an impedance valve to increase volume of air remaining in lungs at end of expiration to improve gas exchange.

G. Subcutaneous emphysema—crackling under the skin upon palpation due to trapped air. Typically found in chest, neck, or face.

H. Tidal volume—volume of air inhaled or exhaled with each breath

II

ANATOMY AND PHYSIOLOGY REVIEW

A. Airway structures

1. Upper airway: nasopharynx, oropharynx, larynx (above the vocal cords)

2. Lower airway: larynx (below the vocal cords), trachea, bronchi, alveoli

B. Ventilation and respiration

    1. Ventilation is the mechanical process that moves air in and out of the lungs.

        i.   Inspiration—the active process of ventilation (requires energy)

        ii. Exhalation—the passive process of ventilation

    2. Internal and external respiration

        i.   External respiration—movement of oxygen from the alveoli into the bloodstream and movement of CO_2 from the blood stream to the alveoli

        ii. Internal respiration—the exchange of gases (O_2 and CO_2) between the bloodstream and the tissues in the body

    3. Tidal volume—normal adult tidal volume is about 500 mL.

    4. Minute volume—respiratory rate x tidal volume

III. GENERAL SIGNS AND SYMPTOMS OF RESPIRATORY COMPROMISE

A. Positional breathing, such as tripod breathing

B. Skin color changes, such as cyanosis

C. ALOC

D. Difficulty speaking full sentences

E. Difficulty breathing

F. Accessory muscle use, e.g., nasal flaring, intercostal retractions, tracheal tugging

G. Abnormal respiratory rate or tidal volume

H. SpO_2 below 95%

I. Abnormal lung sounds

IV. GENERAL MANAGEMENT OF RESPIRATORY COMPROMISE

A. Manage ABCs as indicated.

B. Monitor SpO_2.

C. Monitor $ETCO_2$ as indicated.

D. Monitor ECG.

E. Provide supplemental oxygen if hypoxia suspected and as indicated to maintain SpO_2 of at least 95%.

F. IV access, as indicated.

G. Support ventilations as indicated (adjust rate of ventilations to target $ETCO_2$ of 35–45 mmHg).

H. Consider causes, e.g., various respiratory or cardiac problems, trauma, sepsis, etc.

I. Consider CPAP as indicated.

J. Consider pharmacologic interventions as indicated.

K. Transport.

V. SPECIFIC RESPIRATORY EMERGENCIES

A. Foreign body airway obstruction (FBAO)

    1. Follow current American Heart Association Basic Life Support guidelines for complete or nearly complete obstruction.

        i. Conscious adults and children—conscious abdominal thrusts until the obstruction is relieved or the patient becomes unconscious.

        ii. Conscious infant—alternating back blows and chest thrusts until the obstruction is relieved or the patient becomes unconscious.

        iii. Unconscious patient—CPR

B. Acute respiratory distress syndrome (ARDS)

    1. ARDS is a form of pulmonary edema *not* caused by poor left ventricular function. There are many causes, including sepsis, trauma, OD, drowning, and toxic inhalation.

    2. Signs and symptoms

        i.   Progressive decline in respiratory status

> **Note:** Acute onset respiratory failure in healthy patient may indicate high-altitude pulmonary edema (HAPE).

        ii.   Dyspnea

        iii.   ALOC, such as agitation, confusion

        iv.   Fatigue

        v.   Pulmonary edema (rales bilaterally)

        vi.   Tachypnea

        vii.   Tachycardia

        viii. Possible cyanosis

        ix.   Low SpO_2

    3. Management

        i.   See General Management of Respiratory Compromise with emphasis on:

           ➤ monitoring SpO_2

           ➤ positioning patient upright, legs dangling

           ➤ descending rapidly to lower altitude if HAPE suspected

           ➤ considering CPAP with PEEP

C. Chronic obstructive pulmonary disease (COPD)

    1. Pathophysiology

        i.   Slowly progressive respiratory disease with high mortality rates

        ii.   Includes emphysema and chronic bronchitis

        iii.   Typically caused by smoking and environmental toxins

2. Signs and symptoms

    i.   Possible history of smoking or exposure to cigarette smoke

    ii.   Cough with increased mucus production

    iii.   Air trapping with prolonged expiratory phase

    iv.   Signs of right heart failure, including JVD and pedal edema

    v.   Chronic dyspnea, worsening on exertion

    vi.   Tachypnea

    vii.   Accessory muscle use

    viii.   Possible flushed or cyanotic skin

    ix.   Pursed-lip breathing

    x.   Low SpO_2

    xi.   Abnormal lung sounds, such as diminished rhonchi

    xii.   Clubbing of the fingers

3. Management

    i.   See General Management of Respiratory Compromise

    ii.   Special considerations:

       ➤ COPD patients may have chronically low SpO_2; target oxygen administration to an SpO_2 of about 95%.

       ➤ Only a small percentage of COPD patients are on a hypoxic drive. Do *not* withhold oxygen from COPD patient with signs of hypoxia and monitor respiratory effort, rate, and tidal volume carefully.

       ➤ Bronchodilators such as albuterol or ipratropium are likely indicated.

       ➤ CPAP may help avoid progression to respiratory failure and need for intubation or bag-valve-mask ventilation.

D. Asthma

1. Pathophysiology

    i.   Chronic inflammatory airway disease

    ii.   Death rates rising, not falling

     iii. About half of all asthma deaths occur before reaching the hospital.

     iv. Triggers include allergens, exercise, foods, stress, and medications.

2. Signs and symptoms

     i. Dyspnea

     ii. Wheezing

     iii. Cough

     iv. Pulsus paradoxus (drop in systolic BP of at least 10 mmHg during inspiration)

     v. Tachypnea

     vi. Tachycardia

     vii. Low SpO_2

3. Management

     i. See General Management of Respiratory Compromise

     ii. Special considerations:

        ➤ Monitor peak expiratory flow rates (PEFR) if possible.

        ➤ Aggressive use of bronchodilator medications (such as albuterol and ipratropium) are indicated to reverse bronchospasm.

4. Status asthmaticus

     i. Severe, prolonged asthma attack not reversible with bronchodilator medications

     ii. Bronchoconstriction can be severe enough to cause absent lung sounds.

     iii. Respiratory arrest is often imminent, so aggressive treatment and rapid transport are indicated.

E. Pneumonia

    1. A lung infection, often leading to death in elderly and immunosuppressed patients.

    2. Signs and symptoms

        i. Suspect pneumonia in any patient with a history of chest pain with associated fever, chills, or cough.

        ii. Weakness

        iii. Cough

        iv. Pleuritic chest pain

        v. Dyspnea

        vi. Tachypnea

        vii. Abnormal lung sounds

    3. Management

        i. See General Management of Respiratory Compromise.

        ii. Dehydration is common, consider need for IV fluids.

F. Pulmonary embolism

EMBOLISM

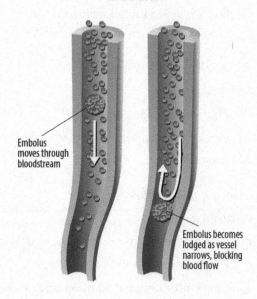

Embolus moves through bloodstream

Embolus becomes lodged as vessel narrows, blocking blood flow

1. Pathophysiology

    i. Blockage (such as air, blood clot, amniotic fluid) in a pulmonary artery that decreases blood flow, leading to potentially fatal hypoxemia

    ii. Risk factors

        ➤ Prolonged immobility of the extremities (such as a long flight)

        ➤ Recent surgery

        ➤ Long bone fracture

        ➤ Smoking

        ➤ Use of birth control medications

2. Signs and symptoms

    i. Acute, unexplained dyspnea

    ii. Pleuritic chest pain

    iii. Cough

    iv. Presence of risk factors listed above

    v. Tachypnea, often with normal lung sounds

    vi. Tachycardia

    vii. Possible indications of deep vein thrombosis (warm, swollen lower extremity with pain upon palpation or while extending calf)

    viii. Sudden cardiac arrest

3. Management

    i. Aggressive oxygen therapy

    ii. Prepare for possible sudden cardiac arrest

    iii. Rapid transport

G. Spontaneous pneumothorax

1. Pathophysiology

    i. Pneumothorax not related to blunt or penetrating trauma

    ii. Recurrence rate is high (50%).

    iii. Much more common in males and smokers

2. Signs and symptoms

    i.   Acute onset of sharp pleuritic chest pain or shoulder pain

    ii. Possible localized diminished lung sounds

    iii. Coughing fit or heavy lifting may precipitate symptoms.

    iv. Tachypnea

    v.   Possible subcutaneous emphysema

3. Management

    i.   Closely monitor SpO_2.

    ii. Supplemental oxygen as indicated.

    iii. Transport in position of comfort.

H. Hyperventilation syndrome

1. Hyperventilation should be considered significant until confirmed otherwise. Anxiety is the most common cause, but there are many other dangerous possibilities.

2. Signs and symptoms

    i.   Tachypnea

    ii. Possible chest pain

    iii. Possible anxiety

    iv. Possible numbness

    v.   Possible carpopedal spasm due to alkalosis and hypocalcemia

3. Causes

    i.   Anxiety (most common)

    ii. Metabolic disorders

    iii. Respiratory disorders

    iv. Pulmonary embolism

    v.   Cardiac disorders

    vi. CNS disorders

    vii. Various medications, e.g., aspirin

4. Management

    i.   Supportive care

    ii. Monitor SpO_2 and administer oxygen as indicated.

    iii. Transport.

    iv. Breathing into a paper bag, breath holding, or other attempts to raise the patient's CO_2 levels are *not* recommended.

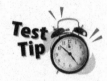

Use the information in this book to create flashcards for items that meet the following two criteria:

    1. Important information you expect to see on the exam

    2. Information you need more work on before the exam

Neurology

I. TERMS TO KNOW

A. Ataxia—difficulty with coordinated movement

B. Decerebrate posturing—arms and legs extended

C. Decorticate posturing—arms flexed, legs extended

D. Dysphagia—difficulty swallowing

E. Hemiparesis—unilateral (one-sided) weakness

F. Hemiplegia—unilateral paralysis

G. Nystagmus—involuntary eye movement

H. Wernicke's encephalopathy—brain damage due to a lack of vitamin B1

II. ANATOMY AND PHYSIOLOGY REVIEW

A. Central nervous system (CNS)

   1. Brain

     i. Command and control of nervous system

     ii. Parts of the brain

       ➤ Cerebrum—largest part of brain. Controls thought, learning, memory, senses. Two hemispheres joined by corpus callosum.

> Cerebellum—coordinates voluntary movement, fine motor function, balance.

> Diencephalon—includes thalamus, hypothalamus, limbic system. Controls thermoregulation, sleep, emotions, much of autonomic nervous system.

> Brain stem—midbrain, pons, medulla. Controls essential functions.

2. Spinal cord (bridges brain and peripheral nervous system)

3. Meninges

   i. Protective membrane covering CNS

   ii. Three layers: dura (outer), arachnoid (middle), pia (inner)

B. Peripheral nervous system (PNS)

1. All nervous system structures outside CNS

   i. Cranial and peripheral nerves

   ii. Sends info to CNS and carries out orders from CNS

2. Two divisions

   i. Sensory division—sends sensory info to CNS

   ii. Motor division—receives motor commands from CNS

   > Somatic: voluntary portion of PNS

   > Autonomic: involuntary portion of PNS

   — Sympathetic—"fight or flight"

   — Parasympathetic—"feed and breed" or "rest and digest"

III. GENERAL SIGNS AND SYMPTOMS OF NERVOUS SYSTEM EMERGENCIES

A. Altered mentation (This is frequently the hallmark characteristic of a neurological medical emergency.)

B. Abnormal vitals, such as irregular respirations

C. Cognitive, speech, motor or sensory deficits (such as weakness, paralysis, slurred speech, confusion, etc.)

D. Posturing (decorticate, decerebrate)

E. Signs of increased intracranial pressure (ICP)

   1. Cushing's reflex: systolic hypertension, bradycardia, irregular breathing

   2. Posturing: decorticate or decerebrate

IV. GENERAL MANAGEMENT OF NEUROLOGIC EMERGENCIES

A. Manage ABCs as indicated.

B. Monitor SpO_2 (target at least 95%) and $ETCO_2$ (target 35mmHg).

C. Do *not* hyperventilate.

D. Aggressively correct and avoid even transient episodes of hypoxia or hypotension.

E. Monitor ECG.

F. Assess blood glucose and manage as indicated.

G. Provide supplemental oxygen as indicated to maintain SpO_2 of at least 95%.

H. Support ventilations as needed to maintain $ETCO_2$ of 35–45 mmHg.

I. IV access, as indicated.

J. Consider causes (AEIOU-TIPS).

K. Rapid transport to appropriate facility as indicated.

V. **SPECIFIC NEUROLOGIC EMERGENCIES**

A. Altered mental status

1. Common causes (AEIOU-TIPS)

   i.   **A**cidosis, alcohol

   ii. **E**pilepsy

   iii. **I**nfection

   iv. **O**verdose

   v.   **U**remia (blood infection, often kidney related)

   vi. **T**rauma, toxins, tumor

   vii. **I**nsulin

   viii.**P**sychological, poison

   ix. **S**troke, seizures, shock

2. Use possible causes and patient history as clues to what assessment and interventions are needed (SpO_2, blood glucose, possible trauma, seizure hx, etc.).

3. Certain interventions should be at least considered for all patients with altered mentation.

   i.   Are spinal precautions indicated?

   ii. Is supplemental oxygen indicated?

   iii. Is dextrose or thiamine indicated?

   iv. Is naloxone indicated?

   v.   Is rapid transport to a specialty facility indicated?

Glasgow Coma Scale (GCS)

Eye opening	Spontaneous	4
	To speech	3
	To pain	2
	None	1
Verbal response	Alert and oriented	5
	Confused	4
	Inappropriate	3
	Incomprehensible	2
	None	1

Motor response	Obeys commands	6
	Localizes pain	5
	Withdraws from pain	4
	Abnormal flexion	3
	Abnormal extension	2
	None	1
	Total Score:	Min. 3/Max. 15

Note: A lower GCS score indicates a higher likelihood of neurological impairment and the need for rapid intervention and transport.

B. Stroke

    1. Causes—ischemia (occlusion, embolus, thrombus) and hemorrhage

    2. Signs and symptoms of stroke

        i.   Altered mentation (confusion, coma)

        ii. Slurred speech

        iii. Dysphagia

        iv. Aphasia

        v.   Facial droop

        vi. Unilateral weakness or paralysis

        vii. Ataxia

    3. Stroke scales/scoring systems

        i.   Los Angeles Prehospital Stroke Screen

           ➤ Assesses blood glucose, facial droop, grip strength, arm drift

        ii. Cincinnati Prehospital Stroke Scale

           ➤ Assesses speech, facial droop, arm drift

           ➤ Any abnormality in above assessments indicates likelihood of stroke.

    4. Management of suspected stroke

        i.   See General Management of Neurologic Emergencies.

        ii. Perform stroke assessment per local protocol.

        iii. Protect paralyzed patient from further harm.

        iv. Rapid transport to stroke center (per local protocol).

C. Transient ischemic attack (TIA)

1. Caused by temporary impaired blood flow to brain.

2. Mimics stroke, but can resolve within 24 hours with no permanent damage.

3. May indicate elevated risk of impending stroke.

4. Treat as possible stroke.

D. Seizures

1. Types of seizures

   i. Generalized seizures

   ➤ Tonic-clonic (grand mal) seizures

   — General motor seizures with loss of consciousness

   — Patient experiences respiratory paralysis during seizure activity.

   — Watch for excessive oral secretions, incontinence, nystagmus.

   — Phases of tonic-clonic seizures

     • Aura: sensation that a seizure may occur. Occurs prior to a loss of consciousness. Not every seizure has an aura phase.

     • Tonic: muscle tension

     • Clonic: muscle spasm

     • Postictal: recovery phase. Patient progresses from unconsciousness to confusion, to alertness.

   ➤ Status epilepticus

   — Prolonged tonic-clonic seizure or two or more tonic-clonic seizures without the patient regaining consciousness in between

   — Typically caused by problems with prescribed seizure medications, such as failure to take as prescribed.

   — Extremely dangerous due to prolonged apnea, acidosis, possible hypertension and increased ICP.

   — Critical interventions include airway protection, oxygenation, positive pressure ventilation, and anticonvulsant medications per local protocol.

➤ Absence (petit mal) seizures

— Generalized seizure with brief loss of consciousness or awareness

— Absence seizures are idiopathic (unknown cause) and rarely occur in adult patients.

— Respiratory paralysis does not occur during an absence seizure.

➤ Pseudoseizures

— Psychological seizure

— No respiratory paralysis and no postictal phase

ii. Partial seizures

➤ Simple partial (focal motor) seizures

— Occurs only in one area of the body.

— No loss of consciousness, but can progress to tonic-clonic seizure.

➤ Complex partial (temporal lobe or psychomotor) seizures

— Patients experience a distinctive aura, such as déjà vu, strange taste, smell, or visual changes.

— Focal seizure, but patient may be confused, have non-purposeful movement, or acute personality changes.

2. Assessment and management

i. Question bystanders when possible to determine onset, possibility of trauma, history of seizures, drug or alcohol use, diabetes, and to determine if patient likely experienced a seizure or a syncopal episode.

ii. Protect airway (no tongue blades, bite blocks, etc.).

iii. Do not restrain patient during seizure, but protect from harm.

iv. Oxygen and ventilatory support as indicated.

v. Spinal precautions as indicated.

vi. Assess blood glucose.

vii. IV access

viii. Consider anticonvulsant medications per local protocol.

E. Syncope

1. Fainting caused by temporary lack of blood flow to the brain

2. Consider common causes

   i. Cardiovascular conditions

   ii. Hypovolemia

   iii. Orthostatic hypotension

   iv. Diabetic problem

   v. TIA

   vi. Head injury

3. Management

   i. Spinal precautions as indicated.

   ii. Supplemental oxygen as indicated.

   iii. Assess vitals, ECG, blood glucose.

   iv. IV access as indicated.

   v. Transport as indicated.

F. Headache

1. Common causes

   i. Vascular headaches, such as migraines and cluster headaches

   ii. Tension headaches

   iii. Organic headaches, such as infections and tumors

Note: Meningitis patients often present with throbbing headache, fever, and nuchal rigidity (neck stiffness).

2. Indications of possible serious condition include:

   i. Headache with associated fever and nuchal rigidity

   ii. Headache in patient over 50 or under 5 years of age

   iii. Complaint of "worst headache ever experienced"

   iv. Headache with signs and symptoms of stroke

   v. Headache associated with exertion, coughing, sneezing, sex

3. Management

    i. Supplemental oxygen if indicated

    ii. IV access as indicated

    iii. Assess blood glucose.

    iv. Monitor ECG, vitals.

    v. Be prepared for possible vomiting, loss of consciousness.

    vi. Transport as indicated.

G. Cranial nerve-related conditions

1. Bell's palsy—sudden, temporary, unilateral weakness or paralysis of facial muscles

2. Trigeminal neuralgia—painful spasms, usually to one side of the face

H. Degenerative neurological disorders

1. Alzheimer's disease—the most common cause of dementia

2. Muscular dystrophy—progressive muscle weakness and degeneration of skeletal muscle

3. Multiple sclerosis—CNS and autoimmune disease. Causes weakness, sensory loss, paresthesia, vision changes

4. Guillain-Barré syndrome—immune system mistakenly attacks peripheral nerves causing muscle weakness. Can cause ascending paralysis starting in the legs leading to need for ventilatory support.

5. Parkinson's disease—chronic and progressive disorder causing tremors, rigidity, bradykinesia (slow, impaired movement), poor balance and coordination

6. Spina bifida—fetal vertebrae does not close properly during pregnancy, leaving part of spine exposed. Nerve damage is permanent, and associated learning disabilities are common.

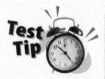

Test Tip

Each question on the certification exam has only one best answer—you just need to find it. The exam (and this book) are based on the current National EMS Education Standards, not state or local protocols. This book is an excellent resource, but it should not be your only resource.

Endocrinology

> **Note:** For information about general management of ALS patients, see Chapter 4.

I. TERMS TO KNOW

A. Kussmaul respirations—deep, rapid respirations

B. Polydipsia—excessive thirst

C. Polyphagia—excessive hunger

D. Polyuria—excessive urination

II. ANATOMY AND PHYSIOLOGY REVIEW

A. Endocrine glands

   1. Hypothalamus

      i.   Located in the cerebrum

      ii. Bridges CNS with endocrine system

      iii. Stimulates release of growth hormone

   2. Pituitary

      i.   Located below hypothalamus

      ii. Releases oxytocin and antidiuretic hormone

3. Thyroid

   i.   Located in the neck

   ii. Stimulates cellular metabolism

4. Parathyroid

   i.   Located on the thyroid

   ii. Increases blood calcium levels

5. Thymus

   i.   Located in the mediastinum

   ii. Promotes development of T-lymphocytes

6. Adrenals

   i.   Located on the kidneys

   ii. Stimulates sympathetic nervous system (fight-or-flight response)

7. Pancreas

   i.   Located behind stomach

   ii. Releases insulin and glucagon

   iii. Normal blood glucose values—see Ch. 5: Electronic Patient Monitoring Technology

8. Gonads

   i.   Ovaries: produce estrogen and progesterone

   ii. Testes: produce testosterone

III. DIABETES

A. Caused by inadequate insulin, which is required for normal blood glucose levels.

B. Type 1 diabetes

   1. Little to no insulin production by the pancreas; aka juvenile diabetes or insulin-dependent diabetes.

   2. Less common than type 2 diabetes, but higher risk of complications, death.

   3. Typically, type 1 diabetics require regular insulin injections.

C. Type 2 diabetes

1. aka non-insulin dependent diabetes (Note: Some type 2 diabetics may require insulin.)

2. Obesity (and likely heredity) increase risk of type 2 diabetes.

3. Far more common than type 1 diabetes, but potentially manageable with diet, exercise, or oral hypoglycemic meds.

D. Diabetic ketoacidosis (DKA)

1. DKA is a life-threatening hyperglycemic complication of type 1 diabetes characterized by extremely high blood glucose levels (typically 400 mg/dL or higher).

2. Causes

   i. May be initial presentation of undiagnosed type 1 diabetes

   ii. Failure to take insulin as indicated

   iii. Physiologic stress, such as infection, surgery

3. Signs and symptoms

   i. Elevated blood glucose levels

   ii. Polydipsia, polyphagia, polyuria

   iii. Decreased LOC

   iv. Warm, dry skin

   v. Nausea & vomiting (N&V), abdominal pain

   vi. Kussmaul respirations

   vii. Fruity or acetone odor on breath

   viii. Incontinence

Note: DKA has a slow onset of symptoms.

4. Management

   i. General management of ALS patients

   ii. IV fluids for dehydration, hypovolemia

   iii. Insulin indicated, but typically *not* administered prehospital

   iv. Rapid transport

E. Insulin shock

1. A life-threatening hypoglycemic emergency characterized by low blood glucose level (typically below 60 mg/dL).

> **Note:** Insulin shock has a rapid onset since the brain does not tolerate a lack of glucose for any length of time.

2. Signs and symptoms

   i. Low blood glucose levels

   ii. Altered LOC (restless, irritable, combative, coma)

   iii. Seizures

   iv. Cool, clammy skin

3. Management

   i. General management of ALS patients

   ii. Dextrose IV or glucagon IM

   iii. Transport

F. Hyperosmolar hyperglycemic state (HHS)

1. aka hyperglycemic hyperosmolar nonketotic coma (HHNC)

2. Potentially life-threatening complication of type 2 diabetes

3. Characterized by prolonged hyperglycemia and severe dehydration

4. Signs and symptoms

   i. Severe hyperglycemia (up to 1,000 mg/dL)

   ii. Diabetic history

   iii. Altered LOC

   iv. Signs and symptoms of dehydration

   v. Increased urinary output

> **Note:** HHS (like DKA) has a slow onset; however, the patient does not have fruity or acetone breath.

5. Management

    i.   Same as DKA (difficult to distinguish in prehospital setting)

 IV. MISCELLANEOUS ENDOCRINE DISORDERS

A. Pancreatitis

1. Inflammation of the pancreas, typically due to gallstones or chronic alcohol abuse

2. Signs and symptoms

    i.   Dull, constant flank pain. Typically worsens if supine.

    ii. Fever

    iii. Jaundice

    iv. N&V

3. Management

    i.   General management of ALS patients

    ii. Transport.

B. Graves' disease

1. Excessive production of thyroid hormones

2. Signs and symptoms

    i.   Emotional changes

    ii. Insomnia

    iii. Weight loss

    iv. Sensitivity to heat

    v. Weakness

    vi. Dyspnea

    vii. Tachycardia

    viii. New-onset a-fib

    ix. Protruding eyes

    x. Goiter

3. Management

   i. General management of ALS patients

   ii. Consider beta-blockers as indicated for a-fib (per local protocol)

   iii. Consider dexamethasone (per local protocol)

C. Thyroid storm

1. Life-threatening emergency, characterized by severe hypermetabolic state

2. Signs and symptoms

   i. Increased stimulation of sympathetic nervous system (fight or flight)

   ii. High fever

   iii. Altered LOC

   iv. Tachycardia

   v. Hypotension

   vi. Vomiting, diarrhea

3. Management

   i. General management of ALS patients

   ii. Rapid transport

D. Myxedema

1. Hypothyroidism characterized by low metabolic state and thickening of connective tissue.

2. Signs and symptoms

   i. Fatigue, lethargy

   ii. Cold intolerance

   iii. Slowed mental function or lack of emotion

   iv. Puffy face

   v. Decreased appetite and weight gain

   vi. Coma

   vii. Respiratory depression

3. Management

    i.   General management of ALS patients

    ii.   Limit IV fluids.

    iii. Avoid active rewarming.

    iv. Transport.

E. Cushing's syndrome

1. Adrenal disorder caused by hyperadrenalism (high cortisol levels)

2. Frequently caused by prolonged exposure to glucocorticoid medication.

3. Signs and symptoms

    i.   Weight gain

    ii.   "Moon-faced" appearance

    iii. Fatty upper back ("buffalo hump")

    iv. Delayed wound healing

    v.   Facial hair on women

    vi. Mood swings

4. Management

    i.   General management of ALS patients

F. Addison's disease

1. Adrenal disorder caused by adrenal insufficiency

2. Adrenals fail to produce adequate hormones.

3. Signs and symptoms

    i.   Progressive weakness, fatigue

    ii.   Decreased appetite, weight loss

    iii. Hyperpigmentation of skin

    iv. Vomiting, diarrhea

    v.   Cardiac dysrhythmias, circulator collapse

4. Management

    i.   General management of ALS patients

ii. Administer dextrose if patient hypoglycemic.

iii. 12-lead ECG if evidence of dysrhythmias

iv. Aggressive fluid resuscitation

v.   Rapid transport.

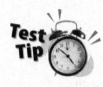

"I Will Pass" Checklist:

1. *Did you previously pass the NREMT exam at the EMT or AEMT level?*

2. *Are you fully committed to becoming a paramedic?*

3. *Have you completed a CoAEMSP-accredited paramedic education program?*

4. *Are you willing to dedicate some focused study time EVERY DAY?*

If you answered YES to these questions, odds are strongly in your favor! This book is designed to help you with step 4. You can do this!

Immunology

I. TERMS TO KNOW

A. Anaphylactoid reaction—reactions that present like anaphylaxis, but are not IgE-mediated

B. Anaphylaxis—life-threatening allergic reaction. Unlike anaphylactoid reactions, anaphylaxis requires the patient to be sensitized, and mediated through IgE antibodies.

C. Antibodies—immune cells produced by body to attack invading substances

D. Antigen—any substance that can produce an immune response

E. Pathogen—invading substance that can trigger an allergic or anaphylactic response

F. Primary response—immune response that occurs when an antigen comes into contact with the immune system for the first time

G. Secondary response—immune response that occurs after development of specific antibodies following primary response

H. Urticaria—hives (red, raised bumps across the body)

II. ANATOMY AND PHYSIOLOGY REVIEW

A. How anaphylaxis kills:

1. Circulatory failure (due to massive systemic hypotension from both vasodilation and capillary leakage)

2. Respiratory failure (due to pulmonary edema, bronchoconstriction, laryngeal edema)

B. Pathophysiology of anaphylaxis

1. Exposure to an antigen

2. Histamine response

3. Increased capillary permeability

   i. Hypovolemia (extravasation of IV volume)

   ii. Decreased cardiac output

   iii. Pulmonary edema

4. Peripheral vasodilation leading to relative hypovolemia (due to massive vasodilation)

5. Bronchoconstriction and laryngeal edema

6. Cardiovascular collapse, respiratory failure, death

III. COMMON CAUSES OF ANAPHYLAXIS

A. Insects (bees, wasps)

B. Plants

C. Foods (nuts, eggs, shellfish, milk, wheat, soy)

D. Medications (antibiotics, aspirin, dextran)

E. Blood products

F. Radiographic contrast media

IV. SIGNS AND SYMPTOMS OF ANAPHYLAXIS

> **Note:** Typically, signs and symptoms of anaphylaxis develop within one minute of exposure, but in rare cases, symptoms may be delayed. Typically, the faster the onset, the worse the reaction.

A. CNS:

1. Sense of impending doom

2. Altered/decreased LOC

3. Seizures

B. Respiratory:

1. Dyspnea

2. Wheezing, stridor

3. Pulmonary edema

4. Laryngospasm, bronchospasm

C. Cardiovascular

1. Tachycardia

2. Hypotension

D. Skin

1. Flushed

2. Urticaria (hives)

3. Swelling

4. Diaphoresis

5. Cyanosis

V. MANAGEMENT OF ANAPHYLAXIS

A. Ensure scene safety, e.g., chemicals, bees, etc.

B. Aggressive management of airway, breathing, circulation

1. High-flow oxygen

2. Advanced airway as indicated

3. Ventilatory support as indicated

4. Treat for shock.

5. Aggressive isotonic IV fluid resuscitation

6. Rapid transport

C. Epinephrine administration IM or IV per local protocol

D. Bronchodilator medications (albuterol and/or ipratropium) for bronchospasm

> *Note:* Can be administered via SVN or in-line during BVM ventilation.

E. Consider antihistamines, such as diphenhydramine, per local protocol.

> *Note:* Epinephrine *first* for life-threatening anaphylaxis.

F. Consider corticosteroids, such as methylprednisolone, per local protocol.

G. Consider glucagon for patients unresponsive to epinephrine.

> *Note:* Glucagon may be effective for anaphylactic patients on beta-blockers. Use in addition to (not instead of) epinephrine. Glucagon may also help reverse bronchospasm.

H. Consider Magnesium Sulfate IV infusion, per local protocol.

VI. TRANSPLANT-RELATED PROBLEMS

A. Infection

B. Rejection

C. Drug toxicity

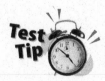

Once you have finished your paramedic education program and completed your study/review plan, try to take the certification exam within 30 days (sooner if possible). Your odds of passing the test go down the longer you wait.

PART IV

MEDICAL EMERGENCIES
UNIT 2

Gastrointestinal (GI)/ Genitourinary (GU)

Note: For information about general management of ALS patients, see Chapter 4.

I. TERMS TO KNOW

A. Cullen's sign—bruising around the umbilicus

B. Epididymitis—inflammation of the coiled tube (epididymis) at the back of the testicle

C. Grey Turner's sign—flank bruising

D. Hematemesis—vomiting blood

E. Hematochezia—blood in the stool

F. Mallory-Weiss syndrome—lacerated esophagus, usually due to vomiting

G. Melena—dark, tarry stool

H. Orchitis—inflammation of one or both testicles

I. Peritonitis—inflammation of the peritoneum

J. Referred pain—pain felt somewhere other than where it originates

K. Somatic pain—sharp, localized pain

L. Testicular torsion—twisting of the testicle

M. Visceral pain—vague, diffuse, dull, cramp-like pain

II. ANATOMY AND PHYSIOLOGY REVIEW

A. GI tract

    1. Upper GI tract: from mouth to stomach

    2. Lower GI tract: from intestinal tract to anus

III. UPPER GI CONDITIONS

A. Esophageal varices

    1. Swollen veins in the esophagus

    2. Usually due to liver damage from alcohol abuse

    3. Ruptured esophageal varices has high mortality rate due to massive hemorrhage, shock.

    4. Management

        i. General management of ALS patients

        ii. Aggressive airway management likely necessary.

        iii. Aggressive fluid resuscitation for shock

        iv. Consider antiemetics, such as ondansetron (Zofran).

        v. Rapid transport

B. Gastroenteritis

    1. Inflammation of stomach and intestine with vomiting and/or diarrhea

> **Note:** Gastritis is inflammation of the stomach only.

    2. Severe diarrhea can lead to hypovolemic shock

       i. Pediatrics and elderly are at increased risk of hypovolemic shock.

    3. Management

       i. Strictly follow Standard Precautions to reduce exposure risk.

       ii. General management of ALS patients

          ➤ Protect airway to reduce risk of aspiration.

          ➤ Administer aggressive fluid resuscitation for shock.

          ➤ Transport.

C. Peptic ulcer

    1. Erosion somewhere along the GI tract due to gastric acid

    2. Signs and symptoms

       i. Often (not always) males over age 50, possibly under high stress

       ii. Often history of heavy use of aspirin, ibuprofen, alcohol, nicotine

       iii. Increased pain after eating

    3. Management

       i. General management of ALS patients

IV. LOWER GI CONDITIONS

A. Ulcerative colitis

    1. Inflammatory bowel disorder of the large intestine, usually starts between ages 15–30

    2. Creates continuing linear, chronic ulcers in colon

    3. Signs and symptoms

       i. Acute abdominal cramping

       ii. Nausea & vomiting (N&V)

       iii. Bloody diarrhea or stool with mucus

       iv. Possible hypovolemic shock (severe cases)

    4. Management

       i.   General management of ALS patients

      ii.   Observe for signs and symptoms of shock

     iii.   Consider antiemetics

     iv.   Transport

B. Crohn's disease

    1. Inflammatory bowel disorder

    2. Can occur anywhere from mouth to rectum

    3. Most common among white females, possibly under high stress

    4. Signs and symptoms

       i.   GI bleeding

      ii.   Weight loss

     iii.   Diffuse abdominal pain

     iv.   N&V

      v.   Diarrhea

     vi.   Fever

    5. Management

       i.   General management of ALS patients

C. Diverticulitis

    1. Inflammation or infection of small pouches along wall of intestine

    2. Signs and symptoms

       i.   Abdominal pain, usually left lower quadrant

      ii.   Fever

     iii.   N&V

     iv.   Hematochezia

    3. Management

       i.   General management of ALS patients

D. Irritable bowel syndrome (aka spastic colon)

   1. Can occur due to stress, or after bacterial infection, or parasitic infection of intestines.

   2. Signs and symptoms

      i.   Abdominal distention

      ii. Abdominal pain and cramping

      iii. Constipation

      iv. Constipation or diarrhea

      v. Increased gas

      vi. Loss of appetite

      vii. Nausea

   3. Management

      i.   General management of ALS patients

E. Bowel obstruction

   1. Can be life-threatening.

   2. Frequently caused by abdominal adhesions, or malignancies.

   3. Signs and symptoms

      i.   Visceral abdominal pain and tenderness

      ii. Signs and symptoms of shock

   4. Management

      i.   General management of ALS patients

F. Appendicitis

   1. Most common surgical emergency encountered by EMS.

   2. Usually occurs between age 10 and 30.

   3. Rupture leads to peritonitis.

   4. Signs and symptoms

      i.   Diffuse periumbilical abdominal pain (early)

      ii. N&V

      iii. Loss of appetite

      iv. Right lower quadrant pain (late)

> **Note:** Pain often becomes diffuse again after rupture.

  5. Management

      i.   General management of ALS patients

      ii. Transport for diagnostic CT.

G. Cholecystitis

  1. Inflammation of the gall bladder

  2. Signs and symptoms

      i.   Right upper quadrant abdominal pain

      ii. Referred pain to right shoulder

      iii. N&V

  3. Management

      i.   General management of ALS patients

      ii. Consider analgesic meds per local protocol.

H. Pancreatitis

  1. Inflammation of the pancreas

  2. Signs and symptoms

      i.   Severe abdominal pain

      ii. N&V

      iii. Possible signs and symptoms of shock

  3. Management

      i.   General management of ALS patients

      ii. Fluid resuscitation for shock

I. Hepatitis

  1. Inflammation of the liver

  2. High mortality rate

3. Often associated with alcohol abuse

4. Signs and symptoms

    i.   Right upper quadrant abdominal tenderness

    ii. Loss of appetite

    iii. Jaundice

    iv. N&V

    v.   Weakness

5. Management

    i.   Strictly follow Standard Precautions to reduce exposure risk.

    ii. General management of ALS patients

V. GENITOURINARY CONDITIONS

A. Acute renal failure

1. Pathophysiology

    i.   Sudden and dangerous (but potentially reversible) drop in urinary output

    ii. Kidneys suddenly unable to filter waste products from blood.

    iii. Typically occurs in seriously ill or injured patients.

    iv. High mortality rate (about 50%)

2. Signs and symptoms

    i.   Oliguria: reduced urinary output

    ii. Anuria: no urinary output

    iii. History of shock, MI, CHF, or sepsis

    iv. Painful bladder fullness

    v.   Edema

3. Management

    i.   General management of ALS patients

    ii. Treat for shock as indicated.

    iii. High-priority transport

B. Chronic renal failure

    1. Pathophysiology

        i. Inadequate kidney function due to irreversible kidney damage

        ii. Often due to diabetes or hypertension

        iii. End-stage renal failure requires dialysis or kidney transplant

            ➤ Risks of dialysis

                —Electrolyte imbalance

                —Hypotension

                —Hemorrhage

                —Infection

    2. Signs and symptoms

        i. Altered LOC

        ii. Edema

        iii. History of diabetes or hypertension

    3. Management

        i. See management of acute renal failure.

C. Renal calculi (kidney stones)

    1. Mass of calcium compounds in kidneys.

    2. Signs and symptoms

        i. Severe flank or groin pain

        ii. N&V

        iii. Hematuria

        iv. Painful urination and blocked urine flow

        v. Fever

        vi. Pale, clammy

    3. Management

        i. General management of ALS patients

        ii. Analgesic and antiemetic medications per local protocol

        iii. Transport.

D. Urinary tract infection (UTI)

1. Pathophysiology: more common in females, paraplegics, and sexually active persons

2. Signs and symptoms

    i.   Painful urination

    ii. Frequent urination

    iii. Difficulty urinating

    iv. Foul odor in urine

    v.   History of previous UTIs

    vi. Fever

    vii. Back or flank pain, lower abdominal pain

3. Management

    i.   General management of ALS patients

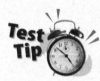

Consider creating a brief (2–3 sentences) pathophysiology flashcard for common medical emergencies and traumatic injuries covered in this book. If you are also preparing for the NREMT psychomotor exam, this will help with the Oral Station also.

Sample Patho Card Front: *Describe the pathophysiology of shock.*

Sample Patho Card Back: *Shock is inadequate tissue perfusion due to a pump (heart), pipe (vessels), or fluid (blood volume) problem.*

Toxicology

Note: For information about general management of ALS patients, see Chapter 4.

I. TERMS TO KNOW

A. Addiction—dependence on a drug that may be physiological or psychological

B. Miosis—pupillary constriction

C. Mydriasis—pupillary dilation

D. Tolerance—need for progressively increased amount of a drug to achieve desired effects

E. Toxidromes—group of signs and symptoms for a specific group of toxins, e.g., stimulants, narcotics, etc.

F. Withdrawal—physiological or psychological effects of discontinuing an abused substance

II. EPIDEMIOLOGY

A. Most accidental poisonings involve children, but are less likely fatal.

B. Adult poisoning and overdoses are less common, but more likely fatal.

C. Most suicide attempts involve a drug overdose.

III. ROUTES OF EXPOSURE

A. Ingestion

B. Inhalation

C. Injection

D. Surface absorption

IV. GENERAL MANAGEMENT OF TOXICOLOGIC EMERGENCY

A. High index of suspicion for scene safety hazards

B. Remove from source of exposure as indicated.

C. General management of ALS patients

D. Attempt to identify specific toxin(s).

E. Consider decontamination interventions per local protocol.

F. Consider specific antidotes if available.

G. Contact Poison Control Center for additional information as indicated: (800) 222–1222.

V. DECONTAMINATION PROCEDURES

A. External decontamination
   1. Remove contaminated clothing.
   2. Remove stingers.
   3. Decon shower

B. Internal decontamination
   1. Intended to reduce absorption of ingested toxins

Note: These methods have diminished in application in the prehospital setting in many EMS systems.

i. *Syrup of ipecac:* not used in prehospital setting any longer

ii. *Gastric lavage:* limited benefit and high risk of complications

iii. *Activated charcoal:* most commonly used prehospital method of internal decontamination of ingested toxins.

VI. **COMMON TOXIDROMES** (also see Specific Toxins section)

A. Cholinergics

B. Sympathomimetics/stimulants

C. Barbiturates/hypnotics

D. Hallucinogens

E. Opiates

F. Anticholinergics

1. Caused by numerous medications, plants, chemicals

2. Signs and symptoms

i. "hot as hades"

ii. "blind as a bat"

iii. "dry as a bone"

iv. "red as a beet"

v. "mad as a hatter"

G. Marijuana and cannabis

1. Can be smoked or consumed.

2. Can produce euphoria, relaxation, heightened sensory perception, laughter, increased appetite, dilated pupils.

H. Huffing agents

1. Examples: metallic paint, paint thinner, Super Glue

2. Can cause cardiovascular collapse, ventricular dysrhythmias, seizures.

 VII. **SPECIFIC TOXINS**

A. Carbon monoxide

1. Signs and symptoms

    i.   SpCO above 5% in nonsmokers and 10% in smokers

    ii. Fatigue

    iii. Headache

    iv. Dizziness

    v.   Nausea & vomiting (N&V)

    vi. Confusion

    vii. Coma

    viii. Dyspnea

    ix. Chest pain

    x.   Cardiac dysrhythmias

    xi. Seizures

2. Management

    i.   Remove patient from source of CO as safety permits.

    ii. General management of ALS patients

    iii. *Must* administer high-concentration oxygen

    iv. Consider CPAP

    v.   Transport to hyperbaric chamber, per local protocol

B. Cyanide

    1. Signs and symptoms

        i. Headache

        ii. Confusion

        iii. Patient may detect bitter almond smell.

        iv. Pulmonary edema

        v. Seizures

        vi. Coma

    2. Management

        i. Remove from source as safety permits.

        ii. Hydroxocobalamin (Cyano-Kit) preferred over classic cyanide antidote kit

        iii. Classic cyanide antidote kit

            ➤ Administer ampule of amyl nitrite for 15 seconds.

            ➤ Repeat at 1 min intervals until sodium nitrite available.

            ➤ Infuse 300 mg sodium nitrite IV over 5 min.

            ➤ Follow with IV sodium thiosulfate 12.5 grams over 5 min.

            ➤ Repeat at half original doses as indicated.

C. Organophosphates

    1. Present in pesticides and various nerve agents

    2. Signs and symptoms (SLUDGEM and DUMBELS)

        i. **SLUDGEM** mnemonic

            ➤ **S**alivation, seizures

            ➤ **L**acrimation (excessive tearing)

            ➤ **U**rination

            ➤ **D**efecation

            ➤ **G**astric upset

            ➤ **E**mesis

            ➤ **M**iosis (pupillary constriction)

    ii. **DUMBELS** mnemonic

➤ **D**iarrhea

➤ **U**rination

➤ **M**iosis

➤ **B**radycardia, bronchospasm

➤ **E**mesis

➤ **L**acrimation

➤ **S**eizures, salivation

3. Management

    i. External decon as indicated.

    ii. General management of ALS patients

    iii. Atropine 2–5 mg IV/IO q 3–5 minutes as indicated

    iv. Pralidoxime (2-Pam) per local protocol

D. Cardiac meds

1. Signs and symptoms

    i. Cardiac dysrhythmias

    ii. Hypotension

    iii. N&V

    iv. Pulmonary edema

2. Management

    i. General management of ALS patients

    ii. Be prepared to initiate external cardiac pacing.

    iii. Consider IV calcium for calcium channel blocker OD.

    iv. Consider glucagon for beta-blocker OD.

E. Caustics (acids and alkalis)

1. Present in many household cleaners

2. Signs and symptoms

    i. Burns

    ii. Dyspnea

   iii. Stridor

   iv. N&V

   v. Hemorrhage

   vi. Shock

3. Management

   i. General management of ALS patients

Note: Activated charcoal is not indicated.

F. Hydrocarbons

   1. Found in kerosene, turpentine, mineral oil, lubricants, paint, glue, etc.

   2. Signs and symptoms

      i. Burns

      ii. Dyspnea

      iii. Wheezing

      iv. Headache

      v. Dizziness

      vi. Cardiac dysrhythmias

   3. Management

      i. General management of ALS patients

Note: Most hydrocarbon exposures are not serious if asymptomatic.

G. Cyclic antidepressants

   1. Not as widely used now due to narrow therapeutic window. Includes amitriptyline (Elavil), doxepin, amoxapine, and nortriptyline.

   2. Signs and symptoms

      i. Blurred vision

      ii. Confusion

      iii. Respiratory depression

iv. Seizures

v. Tachycardia

vi. Hypotension

vii. Cardiac dysrhythmias (esp. heart block, wide QRS tachycardias)

3. Management

   i. General management of ALS patients

   ii. Continuous ECG monitoring (high risk of death due to dysrhythmias)

   iii. Consider IV sodium bicarbonate per local protocol

H. Monoamine Oxidase (MAO) Inhibitors

1. Used to treat depression, OCD. Not widely used any longer due to risks.

2. Signs and symptoms

   i. Hypertension or hypotension

   ii. Bradycardia or tachycardia

   iii. Hyperthermia

   iv. Headache

   v. Restlessness, agitation

   vi. Coma

3. Management

   i. General management of ALS patients

   ii. Benzodiazepines for seizures per local protocol

I. Lithium

1. Commonly used for treatment of bipolar disorder. Has a narrow therapeutic index.

2. Signs and symptoms

   i. Confusion

   ii. Thirst

   iii. N&V

    iv. Tremors

    v. Bradycardia

    vi. Cardiac dysrhythmias

    vii. Seizures

    viii. Coma

3. Management

    i. General management of ALS patients

> *Note:* Activated charcoal is not indicated.

J. Aspirin

  1. Signs and symptoms

    i. Tachypnea

    ii. Hyperthermia

    iii. ALOC

    iv. Coma

    v. Cardiac dysrhythmias

    vi. N&V

    vii. Pulmonary edema

  2. Management

    i. General management of ALS patients

    ii. Consider activated charcoal per local protocol.

    iii. Consider IV fluid resuscitation for symptomatic patients.

K. Acetaminophen (Tylenol)

  1. Signs and symptoms

    i. Fatigue

    ii. N&V

    iii. Abdominal pain

    iv. Liver damage

2. Management

    i.   General management of ALS patients

    ii. Transport for possible N-acetylcysteine (NAC) administration

> ***Note:*** Concomitant use of activated charcoal and NAC not recommended.

L. Food poisoning

  1. Signs and symptoms

    i.   N&V

    ii. Diarrhea

    iii. Abdominal pain

  2. Management

    i.   General management of ALS patients

    ii. Treat for hypovolemia as indicated.

    iii. Consider antiemetics.

 VIII. COMMONLY ABUSED DRUGS

A. Alcohol

  1. Signs and symptoms

    i.   CNS depression

    ii. Slurred speech

    iii. Impaired judgment

    iv. Unsteady gait

    v.   N&V

  2. Alcohol withdrawal syndrome

    i.   High mortality rate from seizures, delirium tremens

    ii. Can last up to one week

    iii. Seizures possible first 24 to 36 hours

      iv. Delirium tremens (DTs) possible second to third day of withdrawal

         ➤ Decreased LOC

         ➤ Hallucinations

         ➤ Tremors

         ➤ N&V

3. Management

    i. General management of ALS patients

    ii. Consider thiamine.

    iii. Consider dextrose for hypoglycemia.

    iv. Consider benzodiazepines for DTs to prevent seizures.

    v. Benzodiazepines for seizures

B. Methyl alcohol

1. aka wood alcohol and methanol

2. Present in antifreeze, paints, paint remover, windshield washer fluid

3. Abused as a substitute for drinking alcohol (ethanol).

4. Signs and symptoms (12–71 hrs after ingestion)

    i. ALOC

    ii. N&V

    iii. Headache

    iv. Dizziness

    v. Abdominal pain

    vi. Blurred vision

    vii. Tachypnea

    viii. Bradycardia

    ix. Hypotension

    x. Coma

5. Management

    i.   General management of ALS patients

    ii. Be alert for hypoglycemia. Dextrose as indicated.

    iii. Activated charcoal *not* indicated.

    iv. Consult Poison Control for additional recommendations.

C. Ethylene glycol

    1. Found in paint, antifreeze

    2. May be abused as substitute for drinking alcohol.

    3. Signs and symptoms

        i.   CNS depression

        ii.   Intoxicated appearance

        iii. N&V

        iv.   Seizures

        v.   Coma

        vi.   Hypertension or hypotension

        vii. Pulmonary edema

        viii. Acute renal failure

    4. Management

        i.   Same as methyl alcohol

D. Amphetamines/stimulants

    1. Examples: Adderall, Ritalin, methamphetamine, bath salts, Benzedrine

    2. Signs and symptoms

        i.   Hyperactivity

        ii.   Hypertension

        iii. Mydriasis

        iv.   Psychosis

        v.   Seizures

    3. Management

      i.   General management of ALS patients

      ii. Benzodiazepines for seizures

E. Barbiturates

    1. Examples: thiopental, phenobarbital

    2. Signs and symptoms

      i.   Decreased LOC, coma

      ii. Slurred speech

      iii. Nystagmus

      iv. Hypotension

      v.   Respiratory depression

    3. Management

      i.   General management of ALS patients

F. Benzodiazepines

    1. Examples: Valium, Xanax, Ativan

    2. Signs and symptoms

      i.   ALOC

      ii. Slurred speech

      iii. Cardiac dysrhythmias

    3. Management

      i.   General management of ALS patients

      ii. Consider activated charcoal.

G. Cocaine

    1. Signs and symptoms

      i.   Euphoria

      ii. Tachycardia

      iii. Cardiac dysrhythmias

      iv. Mydriasis

       v.   Hyperactivity

      vi.   Hypertension

    vii.   Anxiety

   viii.   Seizures

  2. Management

      i.   General management of ALS patients

     ii.   Benzodiazepines for seizures

H. Hallucinogens

  1. Examples: Ketamine, LSD, MDMA, PCP, peyote

  2. Signs and symptoms

      i.   Psychosis

     ii.   Incoherent speech

    iii.   Altered perception

  3. Management

      i.   Heightened scene safety, especially with patients on PCP

     ii.   General management of ALS patients

I. Opiates (narcotics)

  1. Examples: heroin, codeine, morphine, fentanyl, hydrocodone, oxycodone, OxyContin, Vicodin (some contain combination of narcotic and acetaminophen)

  2. Signs and symptoms

      i.   CNS/respiratory depression

     ii.   Miosis

    iii.   Hypotension

    iv.   Bradycardia

     v.   Coma

  3. Management

      i.   General management of ALS patients

     ii.   Aggressive ventilatory support

    iii.   Naloxone

J. Drugs used for sexual enhancement or sexual assault

   1. Ecstasy (MDMA)

      i. Stimulant drug aka: "E," "X," Molly

      ii. Signs and symptoms

         ➤ Stimulant effects (hypertension, tachycardia)

         ➤ Euphoria

         ➤ Increased sexuality

         ➤ Altered perception of time and space

         ➤ Blurred vision

         ➤ Hyperthermia

         ➤ Seizures

      iii. Management

         ➤ General management of ALS patients

         ➤ Notify law enforcement and receiving hospital if sexual assault suspected.

   2. Rohypnol (flunitrazepam)

      i. Potent benzodiazepine; aka R2, Roofies, Rope

      ii. Signs and symptoms

         ➤ CNS depression

         ➤ Sedation

         ➤ Amnesia

         ➤ Bradycardia

         ➤ Respiratory depression

         ➤ Coma

      iii. Management

         ➤ General management of ALS patients

         ➤ Notify law enforcement and receiving hospital if sexual assault suspected.

3. Gamma-hydroxybutyrate (GHB)

   i.   Produces intoxication similar to alcohol; aka Liquid Ecstasy

   ii. Signs and symptoms

      ➤ Euphoria

      ➤ Reduced inhibition

      ➤ Amnesia

      ➤ Respiratory depression

      ➤ Coma

   iii. Management

      ➤ General management of ALS patients

      ➤ Notify law enforcement and receiving hospital if sexual assault suspected

4. Ketamine

   i.   also called K, Special K, Vitamin K

   ii. Potent anesthetic, similar to LSD

   iii. Causes hallucinations, amnesia, dissociative state

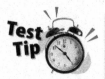

Test Tip

There is no doubt that the certification exam will be challenging. You will intentionally be given questions designed to push the limits of your knowledge. Don't let this stress you out or distract you! Stay calm and focused, and trust your abilities.

Hematology and Infectious Disease

> *Note:* For information about general management of ALS patients, see Chapter 4.

I. TERMS TO KNOW

A. Anemias—Inadequate RBCs. Can be chronic or acute. Can be caused by inadequate RBC production, RBC destruction, hemorrhage, or dilution of RBCs.

B. Autoimmune disease—immune system attacks body's own tissues.

C. Endemic—infectious disease commonly found among a particular group.

D. Epidemic—widespread occurrence of an infectious disease.

E. Erythrocytes—red blood cells (RBC). Transports oxygen.

F. Leukocytes—white blood cells (WBC). Fights infection.

G. Lice—parasitic infestation of skin under hair on the head, body, or pubic area.

H. Lyme disease—tick-borne illness causing fatigue and flu-like symptoms. Good prognosis.

I. Pandemic—disease prevalent over an entire country or the world.

J. Plasma—fluid component of blood.

K. Scabies—skin infestation with microscopic mites that burrow. Spread by close contact with infected person.

L. Thrombocytes—platelets. Bleeding control.

II. ANATOMY AND PHYSIOLOGY REVIEW

A. Components of blood: RBC, WBC, plasma

B. Blood types: A, B, AB, O
  1. Universal donor: type O-
  2. Universal recipient: type AB+

III. HEMATOLOGICAL DISORDERS

A. Transfusion reactions
  1. Causes
     i.   Hemolytic reaction
     ii. Febrile reaction
     iii. Allergic reaction
     iv. Lung injury
     v.   Circulatory overload
     vi. Infection
  2. Signs and symptoms
     i.   Hyperventilation
     ii. Tachycardia
     iii. Sense of impending doom
     iv. Flushing and hives
     v.   Fever
     vi. Chest pain

   vii. Dyspnea

   viii. Flank pain

  3. Management

   i. Stop blood transfusion

   ii. Change all IV tubing

   iii. IV normal saline or LR

   iv. Consider diuretics, vasopressors, antihistamines per local protocol.

B. Sickle cell disease (sickle cell anemia)

  1. Sickle cell disease is one form of anemia. Anemias are caused by inadequate red blood cells (RBCs). Anemias can be chronic or acute. Can be caused by inadequate RBC production, RBC destruction, hemorrhage, or dilution of RBCs.

  2. Pathophysiology of sickle cell disease

   i. Inherited chronic anemia primarily affecting African Americans

   ii. Causes creation and premature destruction of abnormal (sickle shaped) RBCs

   iii. Sludging of blood causes obstruction of microvasculature and vaso-occlusive crisis.

   iv. Increased risk of renal failure, stroke, and sepsis.

  3. Signs and symptoms

   i. Musculoskeletal pain

   ii. Abdominal pain

   iii. Priapism

  4. Management

   i. General management of ALS patients

   ii. Analgesic meds per local protocol

C. Leukemia

  1. A cancer of the body's blood-forming tissues

  2. Signs and symptoms

   i. Weakness

      ii.   Increased risk of anemia, hemorrhage

      iii. Fever

      iv. Weight loss

  3. Management

      i.   General management of ALS patients

D. Lymphomas

  1. Cancer of lymphatic system. Includes Hodgkin's lymphoma and non-Hodgkin's lymphoma.

  2. Signs and symptoms

      i.   Swelling of lymph nodes

      ii. Fever

      iii. Night sweats

      iv. Fatigue

      v.   Weight loss

  3. Management

      i.   General management of ALS patients

E. Hemophilia

  1. Clotting disorder causing poor bleeding control

  2. Signs and symptoms

      i.   Extensive bruising

      ii. Bleeding that is difficult to control

      iii. Look for medic alert bracelet

  3. Management

      i.   General management of ALS patients

F. Disseminated intravascular coagulation (DIC)

  1. Pathophysiology

      i.   Coagulation disorder due to deficiency of clotting factors

      ii. Often due to sepsis, hypovolemic shock, OB complications, cancers, hemolytic transfusion reactions

2. Signs and symptoms

   i.   Bleeding

   ii. Hypotension

   iii. Shock

3. Management

   i.   General management of ALS patients

G. Multiple myeloma

  1. Cancer of plasma cells

  2. Signs and symptoms

    i.   Back or rib pain

    ii. Fatigue

    iii. Pathological fractures

    iv. Hemorrhage

  3. Management

    i.   General management of ALS patients

IV. MISCELLANEOUS INFECTIOUS DISEASES

A. HIV/AIDS

  1. Blood-borne pathogen with no cure or vaccine.

  2. Not highly contagious.

  3. Patients with HIV/AIDS require compassionate, nonjudgmental, supportive care.

  4. If exposed, immediately contact Infection Control Officer or seek care for possible post-exposure therapy (some therapies must be initiated within hours).

B. Hepatitis

  1. There are at least five different types of hepatitis. Follow general management of ALS patient guidelines.

  2. Hepatitis A

    i.   Transmitted by fecal-oral route

      ii.   Often asymptomatic and not often life-threatening

      iii. Vaccine available.

  3. Hepatitis B

      i.   Highly contagious blood-borne pathogen with substantial risk to EMS personnel

      ii.   Up to 40% infection rate following contaminated needle stick

      iii. Can lead to hepatitis, cirrhosis, and liver cancer.

      iv. Patients may be asymptomatic.

      v.   Vaccine available.

  4. Hepatitis C

      i.   Blood-borne, often due to IV drug abuse, sexual contact, or blood transfusion prior to 1992

      ii.   Patients may be asymptomatic for years.

      iii. Disease accelerated in older patients or those consuming alcohol

      iv. Several vaccines currently in development

C. Tuberculosis (TB)

  1. Highly contagious, but treatable, airborne bacterial infection.

  2. Signs and symptoms

      i.   Fatigue

      ii.   Fever and night sweats

      iii. Chills

      iv. Chronic cough and hemoptysis

      v.   Weight loss

  3. Management

      i.   High index of suspicion based on signs and symptoms

      ii.   Can remain dormant for years.

      iii. Use approved N95 or HEPA mask.

      iv. General management of ALS patients

D. Pneumonia

   1. Lung inflammation due to bacterial or viral infection

   2. High risk patients/conditions

      i. Immunosuppressed

      ii. Sickle cell disease

      iii. Organ transplant

      iv. Cancer

      v. Ventilator-dependent

      vi. Elderly

      vii. Low birth-weight neonates

      viii. Chronic lung disease

      ix. Aspiration

   3. Signs and symptoms

      i. Weakness

      ii. Fever

      iii. Chills

      iv. ALOC

      v. Dyspnea

      vi. Chest pain (worsened on inspiration)

      vii. Persistent, productive cough

      viii. Fever, tachypnea, retractions in pediatrics

      ix. Rule in possible pneumonia for any patient with fever and tachypnea.

   4. Management

      i. Wear N95 or HEPA mask as indicated.

      ii. General management of ALS patients

      iii. Consider CPAP.

E. Meningitis

   1. Bacterial or viral infection causing inflammation of the meninges.

2. Signs and symptoms

   i. Weakness

   ii. Decreased LOC

   iii. Fever

   iv. Chills

   v. Headache

   vi. Nuchal rigidity

   vii. Nausea & vomiting (N&V)

   viii. Photophobia

   ix. Seizures

   x. Brudzinski's sign: flexion of neck causes flexion of hips and knees

   xi. Kernig's sign: inability to fully extend knee with hips flexed

3. Management

   i. Use mask and place mask on patient when possible.

   ii. Meningococcal vaccines

   iii. Seek medical attention for possible post-exposure prophylaxis.

   iv. General management of ALS patients

F. Measles, mumps, rubella (MMR)

1. All three are airborne diseases.

2. MMR vaccine is about 99% effective and generally required for healthcare workers.

3. Signs and symptoms

   i. Cold-like symptoms

   ii. Rash

   iii. Fever

4. Management

   i. Wear N95 or HEPA mask as indicated. Place mask on patient too when able.

   ii. General management of ALS patients

G. Respiratory syncytial virus (RSV)

   1. Highly infectious, potentially fatal respiratory infection, especially in infants and children.

   2. Occurrences most common during winter

   3. Signs and symptoms

      i. Cold-like symptoms

      ii. Wheezes

      iii. Tachypnea

      iv. Respiratory distress

> **Note:** Assume an infant with wheezing during winter months has RSV until proven otherwise.

   4. Management

      i. Wear N95 or HEPA mask as indicated.

      ii. General management of ALS patients

H. Pertussis (whooping cough)

   1. Signs and symptoms

      i. Cold-like symptoms

      ii. Fever

      iii. Severe, violent cough

   2. Management

      i. General management of ALS patients

I. Laryngotracheobronchitis (croup)

   1. Common viral respiratory infection (especially in children 3 and under)

   2. Not generally life-threatening (complete airway obstruction from croup is rare)

   3. Signs and symptoms

      i. Acute onset respiratory distress

      ii. Stridor

      iii. "Barking seal"-like cough

J. Epiglottitis

1. Inflammation of the epiglottis that can lead to complete airway obstruction

2. Signs and symptoms

   i. Acute onset without recent history of cold-like symptoms

     ➤ Difficulty speaking

     ➤ Difficulty swallowing

     ➤ Drooling

     ➤ Dyspnea

     ➤ Stridor

     ➤ Sore throat

     ➤ Fever

3. Management

   i. Avoid further distressing, upsetting child due to risk of airway obstruction.

   ii. General management of ALS patients

   iii. In the event of complete or nearly complete airway obstruction, positive pressure ventilation may be difficult, but is usually possible.

K. Drug resistant bacterial infections

1. Bacteria and other microorganisms resistant to antibiotics. A major concern of overuse of antibiotics.

2. Examples

   i. MRSA—methicillin-resistant Staphylococcus aureus

   ii. VRSA—vancomycin-resistant Staphylococcus aureus

   iii. VRE—vancomycin-resistant Enterococcus

L. Rabies

1. A deadly virus spread to people from the saliva of infected animals.

2. Treatable with early post-exposure treatment, generally fatal once symptomatic.

3. Clean wound and assume exposure risk anytime there is exposure to saliva of potentially infected animal.

V. SEXUALLY TRANSMITTED DISEASES

A. Gonorrhea and chlamydia

1. Gonorrhea and chlamydia are different STDs, with similar signs and symptoms.

2. Signs and symptoms

    i.   Painful urination

    ii. Urethral discharge

    iii. Fever

3. Management

    i.   General management of ALS patients

    ii. Can lead to sepsis, meningitis, PID, or sterility if untreated.

B. Syphilis

1. Signs and symptoms

    i.   Lesions (can occur anywhere)

    ii. Rash

2. Management

    i.   General management of ALS patients

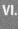

VI. PRECAUTION LEVELS AND DISINFECTION

A. Standard precautions

1. Replaces "universal precautions" and "BSI precautions."

2. Precautions apply to all body substances except sweat.

3. Use appropriate PPE whenever there is an expectation of exposure to infectious material.

4. Appropriate PPE always includes handwashing before and after gloves. Preferred method includes antimicrobial, alcohol-based foams or gels with vigorous scrubbing for at least 20 seconds.

B. Airborne precautions

1. Use appropriate airborne PPE precautions with suspected or confirmed cases of TB, chicken pox, measles.

2. Place a mask on the patient when possible.

> **Note:** Per CDC and OSHA guidelines, tears, sweat, saliva, stool, urine, vomit, oral and nasal secretions pose a risk for transmission of HIV, Hep-B, or Hep-C *only* if they contain visible blood.

C. Disinfection Levels

1. Low-level disinfection

   i. Kills most bacteria and some viruses.

   ii. Use for routine cleaning and removal of visible body fluids.

2. Intermediate-level disinfection

   i. Kills most bacteria and most viruses.

   ii. Use for all medical equipment that was in contact with patient's skin.

   iii. Can use 1:10–1:100 chlorine bleach to water solution or chemical germicide.

3. High-level disinfection

   i. Kills almost all microorganisms.

   ii. Use for all reusable medical equipment that was in contact with patient's mucous membranes.

   iii. Immerse in chemical sterilizing agent according to manufacturer's instructions or boiling water for 30 minutes.

4. Sterilization

   i. Kills *all* microorganisms.

   ii. Required for all non-disposable surgical instruments.

   iii. Requires autoclave or prolonged immersion in chemical sterilizing agent.

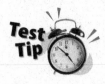

Test Tip

EMT candidates won't get paramedic questions on the certification exam; however, paramedic candidates will get EMT questions. Make sure your EMT knowledge is still sharp.

Behavioral Disorders

> *Note:* For information about general management of ALS patients, see Chapter 4.

I. TERMS TO KNOW

A. Agnosia—inability to recognize objects or stimuli (not due to impaired sensory function)

B. Aphasia—loss of ability to express or understand speech

C. Apraxia—impaired motor activity (not due to impaired sensory function)

D. Behavioral emergency—behavior considered abnormal enough that it requires intervention and alarms the patient or another person

E. Delirium—acute onset of disorganized thought, often due to correctable causes

F. Delusions—firmly held beliefs despite being contradicted by what is generally accepted as real or rational

G. Dementia—slow onset of cognitive deficits. Usually irreversible.

H. Dysphagia—difficulty swallowing

I. Hallucinations—sensory perceptions with no basis in reality, often "hearing voices"

J. Hypochondriasis—delusions of serious physical illness

K. Positional asphyxia—death due to obstruction of breathing related to body position

L. Substance abuse—overindulgence in or dependence on an addictive substance, especially alcohol or drugs

II. PATHOPHYSIOLOGY OF BEHAVIORAL DISORDERS

A. Biological (aka "organic" disorder)

Examples: tumors, infection, damage due to drugs or alcohol

> **Note:** Always consider biological causes of unusual behavior, e.g., hypoxia, diabetic emergency, drugs, traumatic brain injury, toxic exposure, etc.

B. Psychosocial

1. Behavioral abnormalities due to individual personality, unresolved conflicts, coping mechanisms, crisis management, etc.

2. Psychosocial causes are *not* due to substance abuse or other biological or medical condition.

C. Social

1. Abnormal behavior due to social situations.

2. Examples: relationship changes, loss of support system, isolation

III. MANAGEMENT OF BEHAVIORAL DISORDERS

A. Scene safety actions

1. Carefully monitor scene for safety.

2. De-escalate agitated patients.

3. Have an exit plan.

B. Risk factors for potential violence

   1. Scenes involving alcohol or drug use

   2. Large crowds

   3. Violent incidents (such as domestic disturbances)

   4. Patients who are obviously tense or restless, or have an aggressive posture

   5. Patients who are yelling, swearing, or threatening

C. General management of ALS patients

D. Listen carefully and ask open-ended questions. Do not interrupt.

E. Do not rush—these scenes often take time.

F. Be nonjudgmental and honest. Do not threaten or give ultimatums.

G. Maintain safe distance (at eye level when possible). Do not assume threatening posture over patient.

IV. MISCELLANEOUS BEHAVIORAL DISORDERS

A. Acute psychosis

   1. Psychosis is a disorder characterized by sudden onset of symptoms including delusions, hallucinations, disorganized speech or behavior, or catatonic behavior.

   2. Symptoms are *not* caused by schizophrenia or bipolar disorder.

B. Delirium

   1. Acute onset (hours to days) of cognitive problems, usually confusion. Other signs and symptoms may include inattention, memory loss, hallucinations.

   2. Often due to treatable medical condition.

C. Dementia

   1. Slow onset (months) of memory impairment and at least one of the following; aphasia, apraxia, agnosia, inability to plan or organize.

2. Causes include Alzheimer's disease, AIDS, traumatic brain injury, Parkinson's disease.

3. Unlike delirium, dementia is often irreversible.

D. Schizophrenia

1. Significant behavioral changes and loss of contact with reality

2. Patients often present with hallucinations, delusions, and depression.

E. Anxiety (panic attack)

1. Severe apprehension or fear

2. Includes panic disorder, phobias, and PTSD

3. Signs and symptoms, in addition to extreme fear or anxiety, include

   i.   Palpitations

   ii.   Tachypnea

   iii. Diaphoresis

   iv.   Trembling

   v.   Dyspnea

   vi.   Chest pain

   vii. Dizziness

F. Depression

1. Profound sadness that can be unusually prolonged or severe

2. Often accompanied by the following:

   i.   Loss of interest in most activities, pleasures

   ii.   Lack of sleep or appetite

   iii. Lack of concentration

   iv.   Guilt

   v.   Loss of energy

   vi.   Thoughts of suicide

G. Bipolar disorder

  1. One or more manic episodes (periods of elation), sometimes followed by periods of depression.

  2. Manic episodes may present with:

     i.   Inflated self-esteem

     ii. Highly talkative

     iii. Decreased sleep

     iv. Distracted behavior

     v.   Unrealistic plans

     vi. Questionable participation in pleasurable activities with consequences, (e.g., over-spending, sexual behavior, business decisions)

H. Somatoform disorders

  1. Physical symptoms with no apparent physiological cause

  2. Patient may present with the following:

     i.   Preoccupation with physical symptoms

     ii. Unexplained loss of function (e.g., blindness, paralysis)

     iii. Hypochondriasis

     iv. Perceived defect in physical appearance

     v.   Unexplained pain

I. Anorexia

  1. Excessive fasting due to intense fear of obesity.

  2. Patients often perceive themselves as overweight when they are not.

J. Bulimia

  1. Recurrent episodes of binge eating followed by self-induced vomiting or diarrhea, or excessive dieting or exercise

  2. Patients are aware that the behavior is abnormal.

K. Suicide

1. Self-inflicted gunshot wounds and overdose account for over 75% of suicides.

2. Risk factors

    i. Previous suicide attempts (80% of successful suicide victims have made previous attempts)

    ii. Depression (severely depressed patients 500 times more likely to attempt suicide)

    iii. History of alcohol or drug abuse

    iv. Loss of spouse (divorce or death)

    v. Increased isolation, such as living alone

    vi. Loss of loved one, job, money

L. Excited delirium (aka agitated delirium)

1. Causes include drugs (often cocaine) and psychiatric illness

2. Almost all excited delirium patients present with:

    i. High pain tolerance

    ii. Tachypnea

    iii. Diaphoresis

    iv. Agitation

    v. Noncompliance toward authorities

    vi. Tirelessness

    vii. Excessive strength

3. Physical restraint is a risk factor for sudden cardiac arrest in these patients.

4. Aggressive use of chemical restraint medications indicated.

 V. COMMON ANTIDEPRESSANT MEDICATIONS

A. Selective serotonin reuptake inhibitors (SSRIs) (e.g., Prozac, Paxil, Lexapro, Zoloft)

B. Serotonin-norepinephrine reuptake inhibitors (SNRIs) (e.g., Cymbalta)

C. Tricyclic antidepressants (TCAs) (e.g., Amitril, Elavil, Tofranil)

D. Monoamine oxidase inhibitors (MAOs) (e.g., Marplan, Nardil, Parnate)

VI. SPECIAL SITUATIONS

A. Exposure to less lethal weapons (such as a Taser)

1. Patients exposed to less lethal weapons, such as a Taser or stun gun, should be treated and transported unless *all of* the following criteria are met:

   i.   GCS of 15

   ii. Pulse rate under 110 beats per minute (in adults)

   iii. Respiratory rate under 12 per minute (in adults)

   iv. Normal SpO$_2$

   v.   Normal ECG (12 lead ECG when available)

   vi. Systolic BP over 100 mmHg (in adults)

   vii. Dart *not* in eye, face, neck, axilla, groin, or breast (females)

   viii. No associated injury, illness, or psychiatric condition

B. Restraint of violent patients

1. Follow local protocols regarding medical/legal considerations of patient restraint.

2. Methods of restraint

   i. Verbal de-escalation

   ➤ Chemical restraint (examples: Diazepam, Lorazepam, Midazolam)

   ii. Physical restraint

   ➤ Have at least 5 people whenever possible (each extremity and the head).

   ➤ Avoid hard restraints when possible.

   ➤ Secure all four extremities.

   ➤ Do *not* restrain patient in prone position due to risk of positional asphyxia.

C. Substance abuse

1. Pathophysiology of substance abuse

   i. People are not all equally vulnerable to developing substance related disorders.

   ii. Some individuals have lower levels of self-control, which may be physiologically or psychologically based.

2. Signs of substance abuse

   i. Taking a substance in larger amounts, or for longer than is intended

   ii. Wanting to stop using a substance, but unable to do so

   iii. Spending excessive time getting, using, or recovering from use of a substance

   iv. Cravings and urges to use a substance

   v. Failure to meet obligations at home, work, or school because of a substance

   vi. Continued use of a substance, despite damage to personal relationships

   vii. Needing more of a substance to achieve the desired effect

   viii. Withdrawal symptoms, which are relieved by continued use of a substance

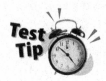

Test Tip

You are at the halfway point! Keep up the good work! Are you on track to take your certification exam when you planned? Remember, within 30 days of completing your paramedic program is ideal for taking the exam.

Eye, Ear, Nose, and Throat Disorders

I. TERMS TO KNOW

A. Conjunctiva—membrane covering the eye and inside of eyelid

B. Cornea—transparent anterior portion of the eyes

C. Epiglottitis—inflammation of the epiglottis

D. Epistaxis—nosebleed

E. Rhinitis—inflammation of the nose

F. Sinusitis—infection or inflammation of the sinuses

G. Tonsillitis—inflammation of the tonsils

II. CONDITIONS OF THE EYE

A. Eye disease emergencies (all can cause blindness)

    1. Central retinal artery occlusion—blood supply to retina becomes blocked

    2. Diabetic retinopathy—damaged blood vessels in the retina due to diabetes

    3. Glaucoma—condition causing increased intraocular pressure

    4. Macular degeneration—deterioration of the retina

    5. Retinal detachment—separation of retina from supporting structures

B. Miscellaneous eye conditions

1. Cataract—clouding of the lens of the eye

2. Conjunctivitis (aka "pink eye")—Infection or inflammation of the conjunctiva

3. Corneal abrasion—painful abrasion to cornea, often caused by direct trauma, foreign body, or contact lenses

4. Papilledema—inflammation of the optic nerve

5. Stye—a red, painful lump near the edge of the eyelid, usually caused by an infection of the oil glands in the eyelid

C. Contact lenses

1. Contact lenses do not usually need to be removed unless there are chemical burns to the eyes.

   i. Hard lenses—remove using specialized suction cup moistened with sterile water

   ii. Soft lenses—remove by pinching lens with thumb and index finger

III. CONDITIONS OF THE EAR

A. Labyrinthitis—irritation and swelling of inner ear. Often causes vertigo, loss of balance, dizziness, nausea & vomiting (N&V)

B. Ménière's disease—disorder of the inner ear. Similar presentation to labyrinthitis, but can be progressive.

C. Otitis externa (aka swimmer's ear)—inflammation or infection of the outer ear

D. Otitis media—inflammation or infection of the middle ear

E. Tympanic rupture—ruptured eardrum

IV. CONDITIONS OF THE NOSE AND THROAT

A. Epistaxis (nosebleed)

1. Anterior nosebleeds

   i. Most nosebleeds (90%) are anterior and minor.

   ii. Bleeding is usually through the nares.

2. Posterior nosebleeds

   i. Posterior nosebleeds are usually arterial and can bleed profusely.

   ii. Blood often drains into nasopharynx and mouth.

   iii. Increased risk of swallowing blood and vomiting.

3. Causes of nosebleeds

   i. Low humidity

   ii. Allergies

   iii. Digital trauma

   iv. Miscellaneous drugs and medications

   v. Deviated septum

   vi. Tumors

   vii. Coagulation disorders

   viii. Hypertension

4. Management

   i. Manual pressure (pinching the nose) for at least 10–15 minutes continuously

   ii. Nasal tampons, per local protocol

   iii. Consider antiemetics as indicated.

   iv. Patient may need cauterization at appropriate facility.

B. Epiglottitis: see Chapter 14 for additional information.

C. Oral candidiasis (aka "thrush")

1. Fungal infection of the mouth

2. Most common in infants, diabetics, AIDS patients, and those taking antibiotics.

D. Ludwig's angina

1. Oral inflammation under the tongue

2. Can develop rapidly and can cause airway obstruction.

3. In severe cases, surgical cricothyrotomy may be needed.

E. Temporomandibular joint syndrome (TMJ)

1. Problem with joint between temporal bone and mandible

2. Pharmacology interventions may include NSAIDS, analgesics, benzodiazepines.

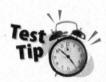

Expose yourself to as many practice multiple-choice questions as possible (try for at least 100 per NREMT category). Use them to test your knowledge and to generate any additional flashcards you might need. Good questions should:

1. be based on current NEMSES and AHA guidelines.

2. include a good deal of scenario-based questions.

3. provide a rationale for the correct answer.

Musculoskeletal Disorders

I. TERMS TO KNOW

A. Cellulitis—infection of the skin and soft tissue

B. Fasciitis—inflammation and infection of the fascia (connective tissue)

C. Gangrene—tissue death, often causing black or blue discoloration

D. Osteomyelitis—infection of the bone

E. Pathological fracture—bone fracture caused by disease

II. MISCELLANEOUS NONTRAUMATIC MUSCULOSKELETAL CONDITIONS

A. Carpal tunnel syndrome

   1. Repetitive motion condition caused by pressure on the median nerve in the wrist.

   2. Causes numbness, weakness, tingling, or pain anywhere from fingers to forearm.

   3. A common work-related condition, e.g., keyboarding, tools.

B. Osteoarthritis (aka degenerative joint disease)

   1. Osteoarthritis (OA) is the most common cause of chronic disability in older adults.

   2. Obesity increases risk of osteoarthritis.

    3. Causes pain, stiffness, and limited range of motion (usually worse in the morning and improves with movement).

C. Osteoporosis

    1. Loss of bone density. Most common form of bone disease.

    2. Asymptomatic until late in disease process, then can cause bone pain, tenderness, pathological fracture.

D. Degenerative disk disease

    1. Typically, a normal age-related degeneration of spinal disks.

    2. Common cause of low back pain, especially in elderly.

E. Rheumatoid arthritis

    1. Inflammation and damage to joints and surrounding tissues caused by immune system attacking its own tissue.

    2. Can occur at any age and usually affects wrists, fingers, knees, ankles, feet.

    3. Causes joint swelling, pain, stiffness, and deformity.

F. Ankylosing spondylitis

    1. Inflammatory arthritis typically affecting the spine

    2. Spine becomes stiff and flexed, causing bent-over walk.

> **Note:** Patient's spine may be inflexible. Do *not* attempt to move spine.

G. Lupus

    1. Chronic autoimmune disease affecting skin, joints, kidneys.

    2. Causes chronic inflammation, joint pain, possible fatigue, fever.

H. Gout

    1. A form of inflammatory arthritis caused by uric acid in the joints.

    2. Causes severe pain, swelling, fever.

    3. Can cause severe pain between foot and great toe.

I. Fibromyalgia

1. Chronic, widespread pain in muscles with tender spots or "trigger points"

2. May be associated with fatigue, anxiety, depression, sleep, or concentration problems.

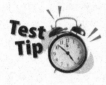

When you make flashcards from practice questions:

1. *Don't make a flashcard out of a specific practice question you missed. Instead, focus on the content that caused you to miss the question. Now, make a flashcard that will help you get any question on that content correct.*

2. *Keep your flashcards short and to the point so you have less to memorize. Good practice questions provide a rationale for the correct answer. If you miss a practice question, look at the rationale and see if it can be used to make a flashcard.*

PART V

TRAUMA

Soft Tissue and Orthopedic Injuries

> **Note:** For information about general management of ALS patients, see Chapter 4.

I. TERMS TO KNOW

A. Contusion—bruise

B. Crush syndrome—systemic complications of a crush injury

C. Dislocation—injury where bone is displaced from the joint

D. Displaced fracture—fractured ends move from their normal position

E. Hematoma—collection of blood beneath the skin

F. Hemostasis—the body's attempt to control bleeding

G. Nondisplaced fracture—bones remain aligned after fracture

H. Occlusive dressing—airtight dressing

I. Rhabdomyolysis—syndrome due to muscle necrosis and release of toxins into bloodstream

J. Sprain—ligament injury

K. Strain—muscle or tendon injury

II. ANATOMY AND PHYSIOLOGY REVIEW

A. Skin

1. Layers of the skin

   i. Epidermis—outer layer

   ii. Dermis—vascular middle layer

   iii. Subcutaneous tissue—fatty tissue inner layer

2. Function of the skin

   i. Protection

   ii. Temperature and fluid regulation

   iii. Sensation

B. Skeletal system (206 bones)

1. Axial skeleton—includes vertebral column, skull, ribs, sternum

2. Appendicular skeleton—Includes pelvic girdle, upper and lower extremities

3. Includes tendons, ligament, cartilage

4. Function of skeletal system

   i. Support, movement, protection

   ii. Blood cell production, calcium storage, endocrine regulation

C. Hemostasis (body's response to bleeding)

1. Blood vessels (especially arterial) will constrict in response to injury

2. Blood vessels retract into contracted muscle (not capillaries)

3. Platelets initiate clotting

Note: Inflammation follows hemostasis (redness, swelling).

III. SOFT TISSUE INJURIES

A. Closed soft tissue injuries

1. Contusion

2. Hematoma

3. Pressure wound

4. Crush injury and crush syndrome

B. Open soft tissue injuries

1. Abrasions

2. Lacerations

3. Avulsions

4. Amputations

5. Bites (risk of infection and rabies)

6. Punctures/impaled objects

7. Blast injuries

8. High-pressure injection injuries (Characterized by a small puncture wound that can cause extensive tissue damage and potential loss of limb.)

C. Crush injuries

1. Compression injury that can be open or closed

2. Increased risk of crush syndrome if an extremity has been trapped for a prolonged period (4+ hours)

D. Management of significant closed soft tissue injuries (RICES)

1. **R** (Rest)

2. **I** (Ice)

3. **C** (Compression)

4. **E** (Elevate)

5. **S** (Splint)

E. Management of significant open soft tissue injuries

   1. General management of soft tissue injuries

      i. Control bleeding

         ➤ Direct pressure (manual or mechanical as indicated)

         ➤ Tourniquet as indicated for life-threatening extremity bleeding uncontrollable with direct pressure

      ii. Splinting as indicated to limit motion and reduce bleeding

      iii. Pain management, such as cold pack (avoid placing directly on injury) and analgesics as indicated and per local protocol

      iv. Tetanus

         ➤ Remind patient to be sure tetanus immunization is current.

         ➤ Booster at least every 10 years

   2. Risk factors for infection

      i. Wound contamination

      ii. Age

      iii. Illness, e.g. diabetes, COPD, cancer, anemia

      iv. Immunosuppressant meds

F. Special situation

   1. Pressure wounds

      i. Caused by prolonged compression of soft tissue

         ➤ Bedridden patients

         ➤ Falls where patient cannot move for several hours

         ➤ Entrapment

         ➤ Prolonged immobilization on spine board

   2. Open neck wound

      i. Apply occlusive dressing to prevent air embolism.

      ii. Control bleeding without cutting off blood flow or compressing the trachea.

   3. Impaled objects

   i. Do *not* remove impaled objects except in extreme circumstances, e.g., impaled object in cheek and unable to control airway or impaled object that will not allow CPR in a cardiac arrest patient.

   ii. Control bleeding with direct pressure around impaled object.

   iii. Stabilize impaled object in place.

   4. Amputation

   i. Manage patient first and amputated part second.

   ii. Rinse gross contaminants off amputated part.

   iii. Wrap part in saline-soaked sterile dressing.

   iv. Place part in plastic bag and keep cool (do *not* freeze).

   v. Do *not* submerge in water.

   vi. Transport body part with patient.

IV. ORTHOPEDIC INJURIES

A. Fracture classifications and common causes:

   1. Linear—parallel to long axis of bone (low injury stress)

   2. Transverse—straight across bone (direct blow)

   3. Oblique—an angle across bone (direct or twisting force)

   4. Spiral—encircles bone (twisting injury)

   5. Impaled—compression fracture (significant fall)

   6. Pathologic—atraumatic fracture (disease, cancer, etc.)

   7. Greenstick—a fracture of the bone, occurring typically in children, in which one side of the bone is broken and the other only bent

   8. Fatigue—stress fracture usually in legs or feet (repetitive activities)

B. Dislocations

   1. Subluxation—partial dislocation of a joint

   2. Luxation—complete dislocation

C. Sprains

   1. Stretching or tearing of ligament, usually due to sudden movement of joint beyond its normal range of motion

   2. Usually occurs in ankles or knees

   3. Signs and symptoms include pain, swelling, discoloration

D. Strains

   1. Muscle or tendon injury due to severe muscle contraction or overstretching

   2. Signs and symptoms include pain, increased pain on movement, usually only minor swelling

E. Management of orthopedic injuries

   1. General management of ALS patients

   2. RICES (rest, ice, compression, elevation, splinting)

      i. Remember to assess distal pulse, motor, sensation before and after splinting.

      ii. Splinting guidelines

         ➤ Splint in normal anatomical position in most cases.

         ➤ Realign angulated long bone fractures per local protocol but *stop* if resistance or severe pain occurs.

         ➤ Do *not* realign dislocations or fractures close to joint unless distal pulses are absent.

      iii. Ensure bandages and splints are not too tight and compromising distal blood flow.

> **Note:** Orthopedic injuries with absent distal pulses require rapid transport.

   3. Pain management (e.g., cold pack, analgesics)

F. Special situations

1. Compartment syndrome

    i.   Ischemic injury caused by increased pressure and reduced blood flow

    ii. Often due to crush injury to leg or forearm

    iii. Signs and symptoms ("The 6 Ps")

    - Pain

    - Pallor

    - Paralysis

    - Pressure

    - Paresthesia

    - Pulselessness

    iv. Management

    - This is a limb-threatening injury, especially once extremity is pulseless.

    - Immobilize extremity at heart level (not above).

    - Isotonic IV fluids may help flush toxins from rhabdomyolysis.

2. Crush syndrome

    i.   Caused by prolonged compression force. Ischemic muscle tissue leads to necrosis and rhabdomyolysis.

    ii. Rhabdomyolysis is the rapid destruction of skeletal muscle due to muscle necrosis and results in the release of toxins into the bloodstream that can cause renal failure.

    iii. Management

    - General management of ALS patients

    - Ensure high flow oxygen.

    - IV crystalloid fluid bolus (to protect kidneys)

    - Cardiac monitoring (due to risk of hyperkalemia)

Note: Albuterol SVN and IV calcium can reduce risk of hyperkalemia-induced cardiac dysrhythmias.

3. Deep vein thrombosis (DVT)

   i. Signs and symptoms

      ➤ Swelling of extremity

      ➤ Pain in extremity

      ➤ Overly warm extremity

> *Note:* DVT increases the risk of pulmonary embolism (see Chapter 8).

4. Pelvic and femur fractures

   i. 95% of hip fractures are due to fall injuries, usually in females.

   ii. Assess for deformity, swelling, tenderness, instability, crepitus, and shortening and rotation of the leg.

   iii. High risk of hemorrhagic shock

   iv. Treat for shock as indicated.

   v. Consider pelvic binder to reduce bleeding (per local protocol).

> *Note:* Traction splints are indicated for isolated, closed, midshaft femur fractures, but do not delay transport of a high priority trauma patient to apply a traction splint.

   vi. Rapid transport to appropriate trauma center

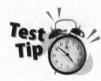

> *The national certification exam is a computer-adaptive test. This means no two people will take the same exact test. The test is constantly adapting to your performance. Once you submit your answer, you cannot go back.*

Burn Injuries

> **Note:** For information about general management of ALS patients, see Chapter 4.

I. TERMS TO KNOW

A. Body surface area (BSA)—the amount of skin involved in burn injury. Expressed as a percentage of total body surface area.

B. Circumferential burn—a burn around the full circumference of an area, e.g., arm, chest, etc.

C. Eschar—leathery, inelastic skin due to full-thickness burn injury

II. TYPES OF BURN INJURIES

A. Thermal

1. Burn zones

    i. Zone of coagulation—center of burn and most damaged

    ii. Zone of stasis—adjacent to zone of coagulation. Presents with inflammation and decreases perfusion.

    iii. Zone of hyperemia—farthest from zone of coagulation. Least damaged area of burn.

2. Four phases of injury

    i. Emergent phase

      ➤ Initial response to burn, e.g., pain, anxiety

    ii.   Fluid shift phase

      ➤ Inflammatory response. Causes massive edema in burns over 20% total body surface area.

      ➤ Peaks in 6–8 hours, lasts up to 24 hours.

    iii. Hypermetabolic phase

      ➤ Increased metabolic workload and caloric demand due to healing process

    iv. Resolution phase

      ➤ Rehabilitation phase and development of scar tissue

B. Electrical

  1. Damage caused by heat created by body's resistance to flow of electricity.

  2. Damage occurs from the inside out, can result in significant internal damage even with little outward signs of injury.

C. Chemical

  1. Caused by exposure to strong acids or alkalis

  2. Strong acids can cause coagulation necrosis to skin (limiting depth of burn).

  3. Strong alkalis can cause liquefaction necrosis, causing much deeper, rapidly penetrating injury.

D. Radiation

  1. Types of radiation

    i.   Alpha—weak. Stopped by skin, clothes, etc.

    ii. Beta—stronger. Travels several feet. Penetrates clothing, first few layers of skin.

    iii. Gamma—most powerful. Penetrates body. Stopped by thick concrete or lead.

  2. Protection from radiation injury (the big three)

    i.   Time—radiation is an accumulative hazard. Limit exposure time and number of exposures.

    ii. Distance—radiation strength diminishes quickly with distance (for example, the exposure at a 4-foot distance will be 1/16th that at a 1-foot distance).

      iii. Shielding—get as much shielding as possible between you and source of radiation.

  3. Signs and symptoms of radiation sickness

      i. N&V

      ii. Diarrhea

      iii. Weakness

      iv. Confusion

E. Inhalation injury

  1. Burn injuries from enclosed space may cause associated inhalation injury and CO poisoning.

  2. Signs and symptoms of inhalation injury

      i. Confined space mechanism of injury

      ii. Hoarse voice

      iii. Cough

      iv. Dyspnea

      v. Stridor (Note: This is a sign of impending airway obstruction!)

      vi. Singed hair

      vii. Carbonaceous sputum

      viii. Facial burns

> **Note:** Up to 80% of fatal burn injuries involve inhalation injury.

III. ASSESSMENT OF BURN INJURIES

A. Burn depth

  1. Superficial (aka first-degree burns)

      i. Involves only epidermal layer and possibly upper dermis

      ii. No blisters

      iii. Causes pain, redness

2. Partial (aka second-degree burns)

    i. Burns through epidermis and into dermis

    ii. Causes pain, blisters, redness, swelling

3. Full thickness (aka third-degree burns)

    i. Burns through epidermis and dermis into deeper tissue.

    ii. Destroys regenerative/repair process and nerve endings.

    iii. No pain to area of full thickness burn, but margins can be painful.

    iv. Skin can be white, brown, red, charred, or leathery appearance.

    v. Leads to eschar (inelastic tissue that can compromise blood flow and ventilation with circumferential burns).

B. Body surface area (BSA)

1. Rule of nines

    i. Useful for large, contiguous burn areas.

    ii. See Rule of Nines table at the end of this chapter.

2. Rule of palm

    i. Useful for small, scattered burn injuries

    ii. Palm of patient's hand = about 1% total body surface area

C. Special situations

1. Circumferential burns

    i. Full thickness circumferential burns to an extremity can compromise blood flow due to edema and inelasticity of eschar.

    ii. Circumferential burn to chest can cause respiratory failure due to compromised chest expansion.

2. Abuse

    i. Be alert for signs of abuse with burns involving children and the elderly (e.g., circular burns, cigarette burns, stocking pattern burns).

    ii. Report suspected abuse to appropriate authorities.

3. Lightning strikes

    i.   Can cause sudden cardiac arrest and respiratory paralysis.

    ii. Do not triage as a normal trauma code due to increased chance of successful resuscitation with rapid defibrillation and ventilatory support.

IV. BURN SEVERITY

A. Systemic complications of significant burn injuries

1. Infection

2. Hypovolemia

3. Hypothermia

4. Organ failure

5. Respiratory compromise

B. Severe burn injuries

1. Partial-thickness burns over 30% BSA

2. Full-thickness burns over 10% BSA

3. Full-thickness circumferential burns

4. Full-thickness burns to airway, hands, face, feet, genitalia

5. Burns with respiratory compromise

6. Burns with associated trauma or those with extensive medical problems

7. Any "moderate" burn in patient under 5 or over 55 years of age

C. Moderate burn injuries

1. Full-thickness burns between 2%–10% BSA

2. Partial-thickness burns between 15%–30% BSA

3. Superficial burns over 50% BSA

D. Minor burn injuries

1. Full-thickness burns under 2% BSA (excluding above criteria)

2. Partial-thickness burns under 15% BSA

3. Superficial burns under 50% BSA

V. MANAGEMENT OF BURN INJURIES

A. Management of thermal burns

1. Local minor burns over minimal BAS

   i. Cooling measures, such as cool water

   ii. Remove constrictive clothing, jewelry

   iii. Consider pain meds per local protocol

2. Moderate to critical burns

   i. Stop the burning process.

      ➤ If skin is still hot to the touch, apply moist, sterile burn sheet until skin is no longer hot to touch.

      ➤ Quickly replace with dry, sterile burn sheet to reduce risk of hypothermia.

   ii. Remove clothing and jewelry that may compromise circulation or trap heat.

   iii. General management of ALS patients

   iv. Keep warm. Damaged skin has impaired ability to conserve body heat.

   v. Apply nonadherent dressings between burns to fingers, toes.

   vi. Aggressive fluid resuscitation per local protocol.

      ➤ Parkland formula aka consensus formula

         —4 mL × kg body weight × BSA of burns = volume IV fluids over 24 hrs (half administered over first 8 hrs)

         —Lactated ringers preferred to normal saline

      ➤ Use caution in patients with respiratory compromise due to risk of pulmonary edema.

   vii. Narcotic analgesia (morphine or fentanyl) per local protocol

   viii. Rapid transport to appropriate burn facility (per local protocol)

B. Management of inhalation injury

1. General management of ALS patients

2. Aggressive airway management and high concentration oxygen

3. Management of suspected CO or cyanide poisoning (see Chapter 13)

4. Rapid transport to appropriate facility

C. Management of electrical injury

1. Heightened scene safety awareness. Assume all electrical lines are live.

2. General management of ALS patients

3. Consider spinal precautions.

4. ECG monitoring due to possible cardiac injury

> *Note:* There can be significant internal damage with little outward signs of injury. Think "iceberg injury"—whatever you can see, there is probably more that can't be seen.

5. Rapid transport

D. Management of chemical burns

1. Heightened scene safety awareness

2. Decontaminate patient as indicated.

   i. Brush off dry chemical.

   ii. Remove contaminated clothing.

   iii. Irrigate with large volume of water (in most cases).

   iv. Remove contact lenses if present and irrigate eyes as indicated with continuous water (do not flush chemicals into uninjured eye).

   v. Chemicals requiring special attention (water-reactive)

     ➤ Dry lime—remove clothing and brush off dry chemical before irrigating with water

     ➤ Sodium metals—water on sodium metals produces heat.

3. General management of ALS patients

4. Rapid transport

E. Management of radiation injury

1. Patient should be decontaminated by trained personnel.

> **Note:** A decontaminated patient is *not* a source of hazardous radiation.

2. General management of ALS patients

Rule of Nines

Area	Adults	Children	Infants
Entire head and neck	9%	12%	18%
Anterior chest and abdomen	18%	18%	18%
Posterior chest and abdomen	18%	18%	18%
Entire left leg	18%	16.5%	13.5%
Entire right leg	18%	16.5%	13.5%
Entire left arm	9%	9%	9%
Entire right arm	9%	9%	9%
Groin	1%	1%	1%
Total:	100%	100%	100%

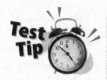

Test Tip

Read each question and all of the answer choices carefully. There is likely some information in the question to help you pick the "most" correct response. You will likely rule out two options quickly and be torn between the remaining two choices. Look for clues in the question and pick the "most" correct answer.

Head and Spinal Injuries

Note: For information about general management of ALS patients, see Chapter 4.

I. TERMS TO KNOW

A. Anisocoria—unequal pupils

B. Anterograde amnesia—inability to remember events that occurred after the injury

C. Battle's sign—bruising to mastoid region (behind ears) indicative of possible basal skull fracture

D. Biot's respirations—abnormal pattern of breathing characterized by groups of quick, shallow inspirations followed by regular or irregular periods of apnea

E. Central neurologic hyperventilation—deep, rapid respirations (without acetone breath found in Kussmaul respirations)

F. Cerebral perfusion pressure (CPP)—mean arterial pressure (MAP)—intracranial

G. Cheyne-Stokes respirations—increasing then decreasing tidal volume, followed by period of apnea pressure (ICP)

H. Contrecoup injury—brain injury away from primary point of impact

I. Cushing's response (triad)—hypertension, bradycardia, altered respiratory pattern indicating increased ICP

J. Decerebrate (extensor) posturing—posturing with arms extended and toes pointed

K. Decorticate (flexor) posturing—body extended and arms flexed; indicates brainstem injury.

L. Epidural hematoma—bleeding between dura mater and skull

M. Intracerebral hemorrhage—bleeding within the brain

N. Intracranial pressure (ICP)—pressure within the cranium

O. Le Fort facial fractures

  1. Le Fort I: slight instability to maxilla

  2. Le Fort II: fracture of maxilla and nasal bones

  3. Le Fort III: fracture of entire face (zygoma, nasal bone, maxilla)

P. Priapism—persistent penile erection

Q. Raccoon's eyes—bruising around both eyes. Possible indication of orbital fracture or basal skull fracture.

R. Retrograde amnesia—inability to remember events that occurred before the injury

S. Subdural hematoma—bleeding beneath the dura matter, within the meninges (above the brain)

II. ANATOMY AND PHYSIOLOGY REVIEW

A. Cranium

  1. Very little space is available to accommodate swelling or hemorrhage.

  2. Any additional swelling or hemorrhage quickly causes increased intracranial pressure (ICP) and reduces cerebral perfusion.

B. Meninges: three tissue layers covering the brain and spinal cord

1. Dura mater—outermost layer

2. Arachnoid—middle layer

3. Pia mater—innermost layer

C. Cerebrospinal fluid

1. Surrounds CNS and absorbs shocks.

2. Created and stored in ventricles of brain.

D. Brain

1. Cerebrum—largest portion of brain. Performs higher functions.

2. Cerebellum—controls balance, fine tunes motor control.

3. Brainstem—midbrain, pons, medulla. Controls many endocrine functions, maintains consciousness, respiratory/cardiac/vasomotor centers.

E. Blood-brain barrier—prevents most substances, such as hormones and neurotransmitters, from entering and affecting the CNS.

F. Cerebral perfusion pressure (CPP)

1. Pressure within the cranium that provides cerebral blood flow.

2. CPP = mean arterial pressure (MAP) – intracranial pressure (ICP).

3. Normal ICP is under 10 mmHg.

4. MAP must be above 50–60 mmHg to maintain normal CPP.

5. Autoregulation: falling CPP stimulates increased cardiac output and peripheral vascular resistance to raise CPP.

G. Spinal column: descending order

1. Cervical: 7 vertebrae

2. Thoracic: 12 vertebrae

3. Lumbar: 5 vertebrae

4. Sacrum   5 vertebrae (fused)

5. Coccyx: 4 vertebrae (fused)

III. TRAUMATIC BRAIN INJURY (TBI)

A. Primary injuries

  1. Focal injuries

    i. Cerebral contusion

      ➤ Blunt trauma to brain causing capillary bleeding

      ➤ Signs and symptoms related to area of brain impacted

    ii. Intracranial hemorrhage (bleeding within cranium)

      ➤ Epidural hematoma

        — Usually arterial bleeding

        — Rapid increase in ICP and reduced CPP

        — Frequently causes loss of consciousness.

      ➤ Subdural hematoma

        — Usually venous bleeding and slow

        — Patient may be asymptomatic for hours or days.

        — Elderly patients and alcoholics at increased risk.

      ➤ Intracerebral hemorrhage

        — Blood irritates brain tissue.

        — Often rapid onset of progressive stroke-like symptoms

  2. Diffuse injuries

    i. Concussion

      ➤ Considered a mild diffuse axonal injury (DAO).

      ➤ Most common result of blunt head injury.

      ➤ Causes temporary dysfunction without substantial anatomic damage.

> **Note:** Patients that deteriorate during prehospital management should be assumed to have something worse than a concussion, e.g., intracranial hemorrhage or increased ICP.

ii. Moderate diffuse axonal injury

➤ Caused by shearing, stretching, or tearing of nerve fibers or minor cerebral contusion.

➤ Is more serious than mild concussion and can result in neurological impairment.

➤ May be associated with basilar skull fracture.

➤ Signs and symptoms

— Immediate loss of consciousness followed by confusion

— Retrograde and anterograde amnesia

— Headache

— Neurological deficits

— Anxiety, mood swings

iii. Severe diffuse axonal injury

➤ Has significant disruption of both cerebral hemispheres and brainstem.

➤ Is often fatal or results in permanent neurological impairment.

➤ Presents as unconscious and with signs of increased ICP. (Cushing's response)

B. Secondary brain injury

1. Is damage due to factors occurring after primary injury.

2. Can be more damaging than the primary injury.

> **Note:** Prehospital management can't reverse primary brain injury, but may be able to reduce secondary injury by:
>
> ➤ Preventing hypoxia by administering high concentration oxygen and monitoring SpO_2 levels.
>
> ➤ Preventing hypotension by controlling hemorrhage, managing shock, and IV fluid resuscitation.
>
> ➤ Maintaining normal CO_2 levels through continuous capnography and avoiding hyperventilation.

C. General signs and symptoms of brain injury

1. ALOC

2. Personality changes

3. Amnesia

4. Cushing's response (aka Cushing's triad)—hypertension, bradycardia, altered respirations

5. Nausea & vomiting (N&V)

6. Pupillary changes

7. Posturing

> *Note:* Pediatric patients may present with bulging fontanelles due to increased ICP.

IV. SPINAL CORD INJURY

A. Spinal concussion

1. Has temporary and transient disruption of cord function.

2. But no structural damage or permanent deficits.

B. Spinal contusion

1. There is bruising of spinal cord with some tissue damage and edema.

2. Usually no permanent deficits, but longer recovery period than spinal concussion.

C. Spinal compression

1. Causes include displacement of vertebral body, herniated disk, vertebral bone fragment, or swelling.

2. Can reduce perfusion, ischemia, and directly damage spinal cord.

D. Cord laceration

1. Can be caused by bone fragments or other sharp objects driven into cord.

2. Leads to cord hemorrhage and edema.

3. Typically causes permanent neurological deficits.

E. Cord hemorrhage

1. Can be caused by contusion, laceration, or stretching of cord.

2. Disrupted blood flow and edema lead to ischemic injury.

F. Cord transection

1. Is partial or complete severing of cord.

2. Can cause paraplegia, quadriplegia, incontinence, respiratory paralysis.

G. General signs and symptoms of spinal injury

1. Paralysis

2. Pain or tenderness along spine

3. Respiratory impairment

4. Priapism

5. Posturing

6. Incontinence

H. Cord syndromes

1. Anterior cord syndrome

   i. Is usually due to flexion or extension injury.

   ii. Often is permanent loss of motor function and pain sensation.

2. Central cord syndrome

   i. Is usually due to hyperextension of cervical spine.

   ii. May be associated with preexisting degenerative disease.

   iii. Causes motor weakness, usually upper extremities and bladder incontinence.

3. Brown-Sequard syndrome

   i. Usually caused by penetrating injury affecting one side.

   ii. Causes ipsilateral (same side) sensory and motor loss with contralateral (opposite side) loss of pain and temperature perception.

4. Cauda equina syndrome

   i. Is caused by compression of nerve roots at lower end of spine.

   ii. May be caused by herniated disk, tumors, infection.

   iii. Can cause pain, bladder and bowel incontinence, lower extremity weakness.

I. Spinal shock

1. Is a temporary insult to cord. Does not usually cause permanent damage.

2. Causes sensory and motor dysfunction below level of injury.

3. May also cause incontinence, priapism.

4. Causes hypotension due to peripheral vasodilation.

J. Neurogenic shock

1. Is caused by disruption of CNS control of autonomic function.

2. Causes widespread vasodilation, relative hypovolemia.

3. Signs and symptoms: see Chapter 6.

V. MANAGEMENT OF HEAD AND SPINAL INJURIES

A. Determine need for spinal immobilization per local protocol. Current research indicates:

1. True spinal immobilization is almost impossible.

2. Spinal immobilization techniques may actually be harmful.

3. Some cervical collars may increase ICP.

4. Immobilization techniques can delay transport of a high priority patient.

B. General management of ALS patients

C. Determine Glasgow Coma Score (GCS)

    1. Adult GCS: see Chapter 9.

    2. Pediatric GCS: see table.

Pediatric Glasgow Coma Scale

	Child	Infant	
Eye opening	Spontaneous To speech To pain None	Spontaneous To speech To pain None	4 3 2 1
Verbal response	Oriented Confused Inappropriate Incomprehensible None	Coos/babbles Irritable cry Cries to pain Moans to pain None	5 4 3 2 1
Motor response	Obeys commands Localizes pain Withdraws from pain Abnormal flexion Abnormal extension None	Moves purposefully Withdraws to touch Withdraws from pain Abnormal flexion to pain Abnormal extension to pain None	6 5 4 3 2 1
		Total Score:	Min. 3 Max. 15

D. For TBI patients, special emphasis on:

    1. Preventing hypoxia

        i. Administration of high concentration oxygen and monitoring SpO_2 levels.

        ii. A single episode of hypoxia (SpO_2 below 90%) drastically increases risk of death.

2. Preventing hypotension

    i.   Control hemorrhage, management of shock, IV fluid resuscitation.

    ii. A single episode of hypotension (systolic BP below 90 mmHg) drastically increases risk of death.

3. Maintain normal CO_2 levels

    i.   Continuous capnography

    ii. Avoid hyperventilation during BVM ventilation.

4. Manage hypoglycemia

    i.   Administer dextrose and thiamine to hypoglycemic patients with suspected TBI per local protocol.

E. Rapid transport to appropriate facility.

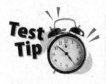

Test Tip

The certification exam is pass/fail. The goal is to demonstrate "entry-level competency." The adaptive technology driving the test is very accurate at assessing competency. If you are prepared and are able to overcome any test anxiety, you should pass!

Chest, Abdomen, and Pelvic Injuries

> *Note:* For information about general management of ALS patients, see Chapter 4.

I. TERMS TO KNOW

A. Evisceration—open abdominal wound with protruding organs

B. Flail chest—segment of thorax moves independently due to three or more adjacent ribs fracturing in at least two places

C. Hematemesis—vomiting blood

D. Hematuria—blood in urine

E. Hemoptysis—coughing up blood

F. Hemothorax—accumulation of blood within pleural space

G. Open pneumothorax—large, penetrating thoracic trauma that allows air to enter pleural space

H. Pericardial tamponade—accumulation of fluid in pericardial sac that compromises cardiac filling

I. Peritoneum—tissue covering abdominal cavity, small bowel, and internal organs

J. Peritonitis—inflammation of the peritoneum

K. Pulmonary contusion—bruise to lung tissue

L. Pulsus paradoxus—drop in systolic pressure of at least 10 mmHg during inspiration

M. Simple pneumothorax—closed pulmonary injury where air leaks into pleural space

N. Tension pneumothorax—pneumothorax causing progressive build-up of air within pleural space

O. Traumatic asphyxia—severe compression of the chest that compromises blood flow

II. ANATOMY AND PHYSIOLOGY REVIEW/ PATHOPHYSIOLOGY

A. Thorax

1. About 25% of motor vehicle-related deaths are due to thoracic trauma.

2. Mediastinum: contains heart, lungs, and great vessels.

B. Abdomen and Pelvic Cavity

1. Three cavities: peritoneal space, retroperitoneal space, pelvic space

2. Four abdominal quadrants

C. Solid v. hollow organs

1. Solid organs

   i. High risk of hemorrhage when injured

   ii. Examples: liver, spleen, kidneys

2. Hollow organs

   i. High risk of infection when injured

   ii. Examples: stomach, bladder, bowel, gallbladder

D. Assessment Tip

1. Always consider the following possibilities for any patient with abnormal JVD:

    i. Pulmonary embolism—expect clear lung sounds

    ii. Right ventricular failure—look for signs of left heart failure (the most common cause of right heart failure)

    iii. Cardiac tamponade—assess for Beck's triad

    iv. Tension pneumothorax—expect diminished or absent lung sounds on the affected side

III. THORACIC TRAUMA

A. Chest wall injuries

1. General signs and symptoms of chest wall injuries

    i. Mechanism: blunt or penetrating thoracic trauma

    ii. Pain, crepitus

    iii. Dyspnea (often increasing on inspiration)

    iv. Bruising

    v. Abnormal breath sounds

    vi. Paradoxical motion

    vii. Signs of hypoxia, e.g., low SpO_2

2. Chest wall contusion

    i. Most common blunt thoracic injury

Note: Infants, children, and adolescents can have chest wall contusion and internal injuries without rib fractures.

3. Rib fractures

    i. Occur in half of patients with significant thoracic trauma (usually ribs 4 through 8)

Note: Fractures to ribs 1–3 and 9–12 indicate high likelihood of significant internal injuries.

ii. Management

➤ Assess for associated internal injuries.

➤ Conduct general management of ALS patients.

➤ Consider analgesics (*not* nitrous oxide).

4. Flail chest

i. Indicates likely associated pulmonary contusion.

ii. Can simultaneously reduce respiratory efficiency while increasing respiratory effort.

iii. Management

➤ Place patient on injured side if possible, or apply bulky dressing to injured side to help stabilize flail segment.

➤ Conduct general management of ALS patients.

> **Note:** The most important intervention for a suspected flail chest injury with inadequate ventilation is BVM ventilation (***not*** a bulky dressing).

B. Pulmonary injuries

1. Simple pneumothorax (aka closed pneumothorax)

i. Caused by blunt or penetrating trauma leading to alveolar collapse.

> **Note:** With simple pneumothorax due to penetrating trauma, air enters pleural space through injured airway structures, not directly through penetrating wound.

ii. Signs and symptoms

➤ Mechanism: thoracic trauma (blunt or penetrating, anterior, posterior, or lateral)

➤ Pain, especially on inspiration

➤ Dyspnea

➤ Tachypnea

➤ Subcutaneous emphysema

➤ Diminished breath sounds on affected side

➤ Signs of hypoxia, e.g., low SpO_2

iii. Management

➤ Conduct general management of ALS patients.

➤ Ensure high concentration oxygen administration.

2. Open pneumothorax (aka "sucking chest wound")

   i. Large, penetrating thoracic trauma causes air to enter pleural space directly through the injury during inspiration.

   ii. Signs and symptoms

   ➤ Penetrating thoracic trauma

   ➤ Sucking chest wound, e.g., bubbling air, frothy blood

   ➤ Dyspnea

   ➤ Diminished or absent lung sounds

   ➤ Possible signs of hypovolemic shock

   iii. Management

   ➤ Apply three-sided occlusive dressing.

   ➤ Conduct general management of ALS patients.

   ➤ Ensure high concentration oxygen and initiate BVM ventilation as indicated.

   ➤ If condition deteriorates, temporarily remove occlusive dressing. If no improvement, assess for tension pneumothorax.

Note: For management of impaled objects, see Chapter 18.

3. Tension pneumothorax

   i. Pneumothorax causes sustained pressure within the thorax.

   ii. Can be caused by simple or open pneumothorax, or positive pressure ventilation.

   iii. Signs and symptoms of tension pneumothorax

   ➤ Thoracic trauma

   ➤ Severe dyspnea

➤ Signs of hypoxia, e.g., low SpO$_2$

➤ Progressively diminished to absent lung sounds

➤ JVD

➤ Hypotension

Note: Tracheal deviation is a *late* sign and should not be used as an early indicator of tension pneumothorax.

    iv. Management

➤ Conduct general management of ALS patients.

➤ Decompress affected side as indicated, e.g., needle decompression, as indicated, and as per local protocol.

4. Hemothorax

    i. Significant hemothorax has a high mortality rate, primarily due to hypovolemic shock.

    ii. Often accompanies pneumothorax, called hemopneumothorax.

    iii. Signs and symptoms

➤ Thoracic trauma

➤ Signs and symptoms of hypovolemic shock

➤ Dyspnea

➤ Signs of hypoxia, e.g. low SpO$_2$

    iv. Management

➤ Conduct general management of ALS patients.

➤ BVM ventilations as indicated, consider PEEP or CPAP.

➤ Treat for shock as indicated.

— IV fluids as indicated.

— Monitor for pulmonary edema.

5. Pulmonary contusion

    i. Frequently caused by deceleration injury (moving body striking fixed object), or pressure wave caused by high velocity projectile or explosion.

      ii.   Signs and symptoms

          ➤ Thoracic trauma

          ➤ Signs and symptoms of shock

          ➤ Dyspnea

          ➤ Abnormal lung sounds

          ➤ Hemoptysis

          ➤ Signs of hypoxia, e.g., low SpO_2

      iii. Management

          ➤ Assess for additional internal injuries.

          ➤ Conduct general management of ALS patients.

C. Cardiovascular injuries

  1. Commotio cordis

      i.   A sudden ventricular fibrillation due to blunt chest trauma, e.g., a baseball

      ii. A leading cause of sudden death in young athletes

      iii. Prompt recognition, CPR, and defibrillation are essential for survival.

  2. Pericardial tamponade

      i.   Compromised cardiac filling due to accumulation of blood or other fluid in pericardial sac, aka cardiac tamponade

      ii. Rare and usually due to penetrating thoracic trauma

      iii. Signs and symptoms

          ➤ Beck's triad

            — JVD

            — Narrowing pulse pressure

            — Muffled heart tones

          ➤ Dyspnea

          ➤ Signs and symptoms of shock

          ➤ Pulsus paradoxus

      iv.   Management

- ➤ Conduct general management of ALS patients.
- ➤ Use aggressive IV fluids to improve cardiac output.
- ➤ Employ rapid transport for pericardiocentesis.

3. Traumatic aortic dissection

    i.   Is almost always fatal within one week of injury and usually due to blunt thoracic trauma.

    ii.   Signs and symptoms

- ➤ Mechanism: high fall or severe motor vehicle collision
- ➤ Significant hypotension
- ➤ Rapid onset cardiac arrest
- ➤ Tearing chest or back pain
- ➤ Pulse deficit between left and right extremities

    iii.   Management

- ➤ Conduct general management of ALS patients.
- ➤ Conservative IV fluids (Mild hypotension may be beneficial.)

4. Traumatic asphyxia

    i.   Severe compression of the chest that compromises blood flow. (usually a primary cardiovascular problem, not respiratory)

    ii.   Signs and symptoms

- ➤ Mechanism: significant compression of the chest
- ➤ Hypotension
- ➤ Signs and symptoms of shock
- ➤ Signs of hypoxia, e.g., low SpO_2
- ➤ Head and neck discoloration

    iii.   Management

- ➤ Conduct general management of ALS patients.
- ➤ Prepare for BVM ventilation, IV fluid administration, and cardiac dysrhythmias.

IV. ABDOMINAL AND PELVIC INJURIES

A. Usually due to motor vehicle collisions with rapid deceleration, crush injury, or compression forces.

B. Trauma is the most common cause of death in pregnant women, often due to abdominal trauma.

C. General signs and symptoms of abdomen and pelvic injury

1. Mechanism: blunt or penetrating trauma, often due to motor vehicle collision

2. Abdominal or flank pain

3. Referred right shoulder pain

4. Nausea & vomiting (N&V)

5. Hematemesis

6. Hematuria

7. Rebound tenderness

8. Guarding (contraction of anterior abdominal muscle)

9. Abdominal rigidity or distention

10. Signs and symptoms of shock

D. General management of abdomen and pelvic trauma

1. Conduct general management of ALS patients.

2. Treat for shock as indicated.

3. Employ rapid transport to appropriate facility.

E. Abdominal evisceration

1. Bowel is most likely organ to protrude through evisceration opening.

2. There is a risk of bowel necrosis due to strangulation or drying.

3. Management

 i. Conduct general management of ALS patients.

 ii. Cover evisceration with moist sterile dressing.

 iii. Cover dressing with occlusive dressing.

F. Pelvic fracture: See Chapter 18

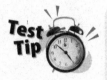

Expect many priority-of-treatment questions on the certification exam. These questions often ask what you should do "first" or "next." Being thoroughly familiar with the patient assessment process will help with these questions. What comes early in the assessment process is generally more important than what comes later.

Environmental Emergencies

> *Note:* For information about general management of ALS patients, see Chapter 4.

I. TERMS TO KNOW

A. Antivenin—an antiserum, also known as antivenom, containing antibodies against specific poisons, especially those in the venom of snakes, spiders, and scorpions

B. Barotrauma—injury caused by changes in pressure

C. Dysbarism—medical conditions resulting from changes in ambient pressure

D. Morbidity—presence of medical problems

E. Mortality—death

F. Surfactant—alveolar substance that keeps alveoli open

G. Thermogenesis—generation of heat

H. Thermolysis—loss of heat

I. Tinnitus—ringing in the ears

II. PATHOPHYSIOLOGY OF HEAT AND COLD DISORDERS

A. Heat generation

1. Increased activity

2. Increased metabolism

3. Shivering

B. Heat loss

1. Conduction—direct contact with colder object

2. Convection—heat loss to air currents

3. Radiation—body's normal method of dispersing heat to the environment

4. Evaporation—dispersion of body heat through evaporation of water or sweat

5. Respiration—loss of warm, humidified air during exhalation

C. Predisposing factors for heat and cold emergencies

1. Age (pediatrics and geriatrics at increased risk)

2. Health (chronically ill patients at increased risk)

3. Medications (many meds interfere with defense mechanisms)

D. Physiological response to heat and cold

1. Cold: typically causes peripheral vasoconstriction and slowing metabolic rate, e.g., pale, cool skin, decreased pulse rate

2. Heat: typically causes peripheral vasodilation and increasing metabolic rate, e.g., flushed skin, increased pulse rate

III. HEAT DISORDERS

A. General signs and symptoms

1. Diaphoresis

2. Warm, flushed skin

3. Increased metabolic state

B. Heat cramps

1. Non-life-threatening

2. Caused by exertion, dehydration, possible electrolyte imbalance

3. Signs and symptoms

   i. Cramps in arms, legs, sometimes abdomen

   ii. Dizzy, weak

   iii. Warm, wet skin

> ***Note:*** Patients will be alert, probably with elevated, but stable, vitals.

4. Management

   i. Remove patient from hot environment and cease exertional activities.

   ii. Oral rehydration if patient is alert with stable airway and no nausea & vomiting (N&V)

   iii. IV fluids as indicated

> ***Note:*** Never administer salt tablets.

C. Heat exhaustion

1. Mild to moderate systemic heat emergency caused by dehydration and electrolyte loss.

2. Can progress to heat stroke if not managed.

3. Signs and symptoms

   i. Passive or active exposure to hot environment, e.g., home without air conditioning or working outside

   ii. Cool, diaphoretic skin

   iii. Increased metabolic activity, e.g., tachypnea, tachycardia

   iv. Weakness

   v. N&V

   vi. Possible muscle cramps

> *Note:* If patient presents with CNS compromise, e.g., altered LOC, treat for heat stroke immediately.

4. Management

   i.   General management of ALS patients with emphasis on:

      ➤ Remove from hot environment.

      ➤ Begin cooling measures (*not* to point of shivering).

      ➤ Oral or IV fluid rehydration as indicated

      ➤ Treat for hypovolemic shock as indicated.

   ii. Monitor for signs of impending heat stroke.

D. Heat stroke

1. Is the most life-threatening systemic heat emergency.

2. Is uncontrolled hyperthermia due to loss of temperature regulation ability.

3. Has the risk of acute, irreversible damage to vital organs.

4. Can be non-exertional (aka "classic" heatstroke) or exertional.

5. Signs and symptoms

   i.   Altered or decreased LOC

   ii. Usually hot/dry skin due to loss of sweat mechanism.

> *Note:* Patient may still be diaphoretic in high humidity environment.

   iii. Core temp usually at least 105 degrees F (40.6 C)

   iv. Abnormal respirations

   v. Signs of shock, e.g., tachycardia, hypotension

   vi. Seizures

6. Management

   i.   *Must* remove patient from hot environment.

   ii.   Initiate rapid cooling measures (target: 102 degrees F/39 C).

      ➤ Perform en route to hospital.

      ➤ Remove clothing, cover with sheets soaked in tepid water.

   iii.   Conduct general management of ALS patients with emphasis on:

      ➤ Treating for shock.

      ➤ ECG monitoring for dysrhythmias.

   iv.   Employ rapid transport.

IV. COLD DISORDERS

A. Frostbite

  1. Superficial frostbite (aka frostnip) causes redness, blanching, and loss of sensation. Little risk of permanent injury.

  2. Deep frostbite

    i.   Affects deep tissue layers.

    ii.   White, hard appearance to skin with loss of sensation

    iii.   Management

       ➤ Remove from cold environment.

       ➤ Assess for possible hypothermia.

       ➤ Do not allow tissue to refreeze.

       ➤ Do *not* massage frozen tissue.

       ➤ Apply dry, sterile dressing and elevate.

       ➤ Transport for rewarming.

       ➤ Consider analgesic meds as indicated and per local protocol.

  3. Trench foot (aka immersion foot)

    i.   Similar to frostbite, occurs when tissue immersed in cold water for prolonged period.

    ii.   Management includes drying, warming, and elevating feet.

B. Hypothermia

1. Is a potentially life-threatening systemic cold emergency.

2. Core temp below 95 degrees F (35 C)

    i.   Mild hypothermia—core temp above 90 degrees F (32 C) with signs and symptoms

    ii.   Severe hypothermia—core temp below 90 degrees F (32 C) with signs and symptoms

3. Signs and symptoms

    i.   Altered LOC (mild)/unresponsive (severe)

    ii.   Tachycardia (mild)/bradycardia (severe)

    iii.   Tachypnea (mild)/bradypnea (severe)

    iv.   Shivering (mild)/loss of shivering (severe)

    v.   Atrial fibrillation (most common hypothermic dysrhythmia)

    vi.   Coma, apnea, ventricular fibrillation, asystole (severe)

4. Management

    i.   Remove from cold environment.

    ii.   Remove wet clothes.

    iii.   Passive rewarming measures, e.g., blankets

    iv.   Avoid rough handling (can induce VF).

    v.   Monitor core temperature.

    vi.   ECG monitoring

    vii.   Prolong pulse check due to chance of severe bradycardia.

       ➤ Patients with a pulse

          — General management of ALS patients

          — Rapid transport

       ➤ Cardiac arrest patients

          — Begin CPR.

          — ACLS guidelines based on core temp.

             (i) Core temp below 86 degrees F (30 C)

                ➤ If VF, defib **once** at 360 J or biphasic equivalent

➤ Continue CPR.

➤ No medications or further defibrillation

(ii) Core temp above 86 degrees F (30 C)

➤ Continue CPR.

➤ Defib and administer meds per standard ACLS guidelines.

viii. Contraindications for initiating resuscitation of hypothermic patient

➤ Submersion greater than one hour

➤ Core temp below 50 degrees F (10 C)

➤ Obvious fatal injuries

➤ Chest wall rigidity prevents CPR

> **Note:** Do **not** discontinue resuscitation of patient that is still hypothermic. ("Patients are not dead until they are warm and dead.")

V. DROWNING

A. Pathophysiology of drowning incident

1. Victim enters water (at least the airway)

2. Breath holding

3. Water swallowing

4. Laryngospasm

5. Hypoxia

6. Airway relaxes

7. Water enters lungs

8. Surfactant washout

9. Cardiac arrest

B. Mammalian diving reflex: exposure to near-freezing water can rapidly slow metabolic rate and improve survival rates.

C. Management of drowning incident

1. Remove patient from water only if safe to do so. Initiate spinal precautions as indicated.

2. Avoid placing patient on surface that can cause surface burns, e.g., hot concrete.

3. Aggressive management of ABC as quickly as possible, while still in water if possible. Prepare for vomiting.

4. CPR and defibrillation as indicated.

   Remember: Initiate CPR for an unresponsive pediatric patient with a pulse below 60 beats per minute.

5. Manage hypothermia as indicated (wet patients lose body heat rapidly).

VI. DIVING EMERGENCIES

A. Gas laws

1. Boyle's law—volume of a gas is inversely proportional to its pressure.

2. Dalton's law—total pressure of mixed gases is equal to sum of partial pressures of each gas.

3. Henry's law—amount of gas dissolved in a given volume of fluid is proportional to the pressure of the gases above it.

B. Diving emergencies

1. Descent barotrauma (aka "the squeeze")

   i. Signs and symptoms

   ➤ Ear pain

   ➤ Tinnitus

   ➤ Dizziness

   ➤ Hearing loss

2. Nitrogen narcosis (aka "rapture of the deep")

   i. Can occur at bottom of dive.

   ii. Signs and symptoms

> ➤ Altered mentation, impaired judgment

> ➤ Intoxicated sensation, appearance

3. Decompression sickness (aka "the bends")

    i.   Is caused by barotrauma during ascent.

    ii.   Signs and symptoms

> ➤ Severe pain, especially in the joints and abdomen

> ➤ ALOC

> ➤ Dizziness

> ➤ N&V

> ➤ Vertigo

> ➤ Tinnitus

> ➤ Chest pain

> ➤ Cough

> ➤ Pulmonary edema

4. Pulmonary overpressure

    i.   Is caused by barotrauma during ascent (usually holding breath during ascent).

    ii.   Can cause pneumothorax, arterial gas embolism, and pneumomediastinum (abnormal presence of air in the mediastinum).

    iii.   Signs and symptoms

> ➤ Chest pain

> ➤ Dyspnea

> ➤ Diminished breath sounds (pneumothorax)

> ➤ Signs and symptoms of stroke (arterial gas embolism)

> ➤ Narrowing pulse pressure (pneumomediastinum)

5. General management of diving emergencies

    i.   General management of ALS patients with emphasis on:

> ➤ Administration of high concentration oxygen.

> ➤ Monitor for signs of pneumothorax.

    ii.   Consider CPAP (*not* for pneumothorax).

   iii. Transport to hyperbaric chamber (per local protocol).

       ➤ Use caution with air evacuation due to possible exposure to barometric pressure changes.

VII. HIGH ALTITUDE SICKNESS

A. Caused by exposure to high altitude, low oxygen environments.

B. Acute mountain sickness (AMS)

  1. Typically caused by rapid ascent to about 6,600 feet or above.

  2. Signs and symptoms

     i. Dizziness

     ii. Weakness

     iii. Dyspnea

C. High-altitude cerebral edema (HACE)

  1. Considered severe AMS

  2. Signs and symptoms

     i. Signs and symptoms of AMS

     ii. Altered mental status

     iii. Ataxia

D. High-altitude pulmonary edema (HAPE)

  1. Signs and symptoms

     i. Dyspnea

     ii. Chest pain

     iii. Cough

     iv. Weakness

     v. Abnormal lung sounds

     vi. Tachypnea

     vii. Tachycardia

E. General management of high altitude sickness

1. Halt ascent; descend if possible.

2. General management of ALS patients with emphasis on high concentration oxygen administration.

3. Consider steroids, such as dexamethasone per local protocol.

VIII. BITES AND STINGS

A. Conduct general management of bites and stings.

1. Ensure scene safety before initiating treatment.

2. Remove patient from exposure environment.

3. Conduct general management of ALS patients.

4. Prevent further envenomation when possible, e.g., remove stingers.

5. Wash area.

6. Cold compress as indicated for pain.

7. Assess and manage anaphylaxis as indicated (see Chapter 6).

8. Contact Poison Control or medical direction for additional guidance as needed.

9. Transport as indicated.

B. Hymenoptera (wasps, bees, hornets, ants)

1. Most bites and stings present local problems only, but can induce anaphylactic shock.

2. Honeybees sting only once, leaving venom sac behind. Other Hymenoptera can sting repeatedly.

3. Signs and symptoms

   i. Local pain

   ii. Redness

   iii. Swelling

   iv. Skin welt

C. Spiders

  1. Brown recluse

    i. Bites are not immediately painful and may not be noticed at the time.

    ii. Signs and symptoms

      ➤ Localized pain, redness, and swelling develop over several hours.

      ➤ Local tissue necrosis can develop over days to weeks.

      ➤ In rare cases, fever, chills, N&V, disseminated intravascular coagulation may develop.

    iii. Management

      ➤ Conduct general management of ALS patients.

      ➤ No antivenin available

      ➤ Transport as indicated.

> *Note:* Antihistamines and surgical repair of necrotic tissue may be necessary.

  2. Black widow

    i. Bites to humans come from female black widow spiders.

    ii. Signs and symptoms

      ➤ Immediate, localized pain, redness, and swelling

      ➤ Muscle spasms may develop.

      ➤ In rare cases, N&V, seizures, paralysis, and decreased LOC

    iii. Management

      ➤ General management of ALS patients

        — Monitor carefully for hypertensive crisis.

      ➤ Consider benzodiazepines or calcium gluconate (not calcium chloride) for severe muscle spasms per local protocol.

      ➤ Transport as indicated.

> ***Note:*** Antivenin is available.

D. Scorpions

    1. Most scorpion stings unlikely to produce systemic complications.

    2. Signs and symptoms

        i.   Local pain, burning

        ii. Numbness

        iii. Slurred speech

        iv. Hyperactivity (especially in children)

        v. Nystagmus

        vi. Muscle twitching

        vii. Excessive salivation

        viii. Abdominal cramps, N&V

        ix. Seizures

    3. Management

        i.   General management of ALS patients

        ii. Apply constricting band (no tighter than watchband) to reduce lymphatic flow (per local protocol).

        iii. Do not administer analgesics; may increase toxicity.

        iv. Transport

> ***Note:*** Antivenin (aka antivenom) is available, but risk of anaphylactic reaction is high.

E. Snakebites

    1. Inappropriate interventions

        i.   Do *not* apply ice, cold packs, etc.

        ii. Do *not* apply tourniquet.

        iii. Do *not* incise wound.

iv. Do *not* use a snake bite kit.

v. Do *not* apply electrical stimulation.

2. Pit vipers

    i. Bite can cause shock and death within 30 minutes; however, most deaths occur 6–30 hours after bite.

    ii. Signs and symptoms

- Local pain, swelling
- Oozing at wound site
- Dizziness, weakness, syncope
- N&V
- Diarrhea
- Signs and symptoms of shock, e.g., tachycardia, hypotension
- Respiratory failure

    iii. Management

- Conduct general management of ALS patients.
- Immobilize bite site.
- Do *not* apply constricting band.
- Transport (Antivenin is available.)

3. Coral snake

    i. Neurotoxic venom

    ii. Signs and symptoms

- Numbness, weakness
- Decreased LOC
- Ataxia
- Slurred speech
- Abdominal pain, N&V
- Hypotension
- Respiratory failure
- Seizures

      iii. Management

        ➤ Conduct general management of ALS patients.

        ➤ Wash site with water.

        ➤ Apply compression bandage (per local protocol) and keep extremity at heart level.

        ➤ Immobilize limb.

        ➤ Transport. (Antivenin is available.)

F. Marine animals

  1. Includes jellyfish, corals, stingrays, urchins.

  2. *All* can cause severe pain and are typically heat-sensitive (heat reduces pain).

  3. Signs and symptoms

      i. Intense local pain

      ii. N&V

      iii. Dyspnea

      iv. Weakness

      v. Tachycardia

      vi. Hypotension

  4. Management

      i. Conduct general management of ALS patients.

      ii. Apply constricting band (no tighter than watch band) to reduce lymphatic flow.

      iii. Apply heat (110–113 degrees F).

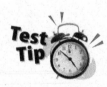

Test Tip

Questions on the certification exam will not contain a great deal of irrelevant information. That means two things:

  1. The information included in the questions is important.

  2. Answer the questions asked. Don't "what if" the questions by putting things in that aren't there.

PART VI
SPECIAL PATIENTS

OB & GYN
Emergencies

> **Note:** For information about general management of ALS patients, see Chapter 4.

I. TERMS TO KNOW

A. Antepartum—prior to delivery

B. Bloody show—passage of a small amount of blood or blood-tinged mucus near the end of pregnancy

C. Braxton hicks—sporadic uterine contractions that can occur prior to active labor

D. Endometritis—infection of the uterine lining

E. Fundal height—distance in cm from pubic symphysis to top of uterine fundus. Each cm = one week of gestation

F. Gravida—total number of pregnancies

G. Hyperemesis gravidarum—severe nausea and vomiting during pregnancy

H. Menarche—the first occurrence of menstruation

I. Mittelschmerz—Unilateral lower quadrant abdominal pain that occurs midway through a menstrual cycle

J. Multigravida—a woman who has had at least two pregnancies

K. Nullipara—a woman who has never given birth

L. Para—total number of pregnancies reaching viable gestational age (live births and stillbirths)

M. Postpartum—after delivery

N. Primigravida—a woman who is pregnant for the first time

O. Ruptured membranes (ROM)—rupture of the amniotic sac

II. ANATOMY AND PHYSIOLOGY REVIEW

A. Maternal changes during pregnancy

1. Airway

   i. Resting respiratory rate increases.

   ii. Slowed digestion increases risk of vomiting and aspiration.

   iii. Increased risk of hypoxia (oxygen demand increases up to 40%).

2. CNS

   i. Increased risk of syncope

3. Cardiovascular

   i. Cardiac output increases up to 50%.

   ii. Resting heart rate increases.

   iii. Significant increase in uterine blood flow, increasing risk of hemorrhage from abdominal injuries

   iv. Increased RBC production, but greater plasma increase leads to relative anemia.

   v. Increased risk of pulmonary embolism

   vi. Increase risk of shock (up to 80% fetal mortality from maternal shock)

   vii. Increased risk of hypertensive emergencies

4. Endocrine

    i.   Increased risk of diabetes (gestational diabetes) or diabetic complications

5. GI/GU

    i.   Weight gain and enlarging uterus cause constipation and risk of supine hypotensive syndrome.

    ii. Increased urinary frequency.

III. SPECIAL ASSESSMENT CONSIDERATIONS

A. Determine if delivery is imminent, e.g., urge to push.

> *Note:* Check for crowning (during contraction) only if imminent delivery is suspected.

B. Increased risk of injury and death due to motor vehicle collisions, falls, and domestic violence.

C. Determine gestational age of fetus, e.g., how many weeks pregnant, estimated due date, fundal height.

D. Provide emotional support.

E. Carefully monitor for signs of hypoxia, shock, supine hypotensive syndrome.

IV. OBSTETRICAL COMPLICATIONS

A. Vaginal bleeding

1. Common causes

    i.   Spontaneous abortion (miscarriage)

    ii. Ectopic pregnancy

    iii. Abruptio placenta

    iv. Placenta previa

    v. Postpartum hemorrhage (under 500 mL is normal)

2. General management of OB-related vaginal bleeding

    i. General management of ALS patients

    ii. Treat for shock as indicated.

    iii. Consider postpartum interventions, per local protocol.

       ➤ Fundal massage

       ➤ Breast feeding

       ➤ Oxytocin administration

    iv. Employ rapid transport to appropriate facility.

B. Uterine rupture

1. Can result from labor or trauma.

2. Signs and symptoms

    i. Severe abdominal pain

    ii. Signs and symptoms of shock

    iii. Possible absence of fetal heart tones

3. Management

    i. Conduct general management of ALS patients.

    ii. Treat for shock.

    iii. Employ rapid transport (for mother and to determine fetus viability).

C. Spontaneous abortion (miscarriage)

1. Delivery of fetus before viability (weeks 20–22 of gestation)

2. Signs and symptoms

    i. Severe cramping, lower abdominal pain

    ii. Vaginal bleeding

    iii. Passage of tissue, clots

3. Management

    i. Conduct general management of ALS patients.

    ii. Treat for shock.

    iii. Give emotional support.

    iv. Employ rapid transport.

D. Placenta previa

1. Abnormal placement of placenta over cervical opening

2. Signs and symptoms

   i. Bright red, painless vaginal bleeding during third trimester

   Note: Treat painless vaginal bleeding during later stages of pregnancy as placenta previa until proven otherwise.

3. Management

   i. Provide general management of ALS patients.

   ii. Treat for shock as indicated.

   iii. Transport for possible Caesarean section.

E. Abruptio placenta

1. Premature separation of the placenta from the uterine wall

2. High risk of fetal mortality

3. Signs and symptoms

   i. Painful vaginal bleeding in later stages of pregnancy

   ii. Signs and symptoms of shock

   Note: Blood loss can be trapped, with no vaginal bleeding evident.

4. Management

   i. Use aggressive management of shock.

   ii. Place patient left lateral recumbent.

   iii. Employ rapid transport to appropriate facility.

F. Hypertensive complications of pregnancy

1. Preeclampsia

   i. Pathophysiology

      ➤ Is the most common hypertensive disorder of pregnancy.

      ➤ Can progress from mild to severe.

> ➤ Increase in systolic pressure of 30 mmHg and/or 15 mmHg increase in diastolic pressure on at least two occasions (at least 6 hours apart)

> ➤ Usually occurs from last 10 weeks of gestation through 48 hours postpartum.

    ii.   Signs and symptoms

> ➤ Hypertension

> ➤ Edema

> ➤ Headache

> ➤ Visual disturbances

> ➤ Hyperactive reflexes

> ➤ Pulmonary edema

> ➤ Increased urinary output

    iii. Management

> ➤ Provide general management of ALS patients.

> ➤ Keep patient calm, dim lights, avoid lights and siren.

> ➤ Place left lateral recumbent.

> ➤ Consider magnesium sulfate per local protocol.

2. Eclampsia

    i.   Seizures due to hypertensive disorder of pregnancy

    ii. High risk of maternal and fetal death

    iii. Signs and symptoms

> ➤ Generalized tonic-clonic seizures

> ➤ History of preeclampsia

> ➤ Are preceded by signs and symptoms of preeclampsia.

    iv. Management

> ➤ Same as above

> ➤ Magnesium sulfate is preferred to control seizures, then diazepam or other benzodiazepines.

G. Supine hypotensive syndrome

1. Occurs in later stages of pregnancy when uterus compresses inferior vena cava while supine.

2. Signs and symptoms

    i. Patient supine for extended period

    ii. Dizziness

    iii. Syncope

    iv. Hypotension

3. Management

    i. Place patient left lateral recumbent (usually sufficient).

    ii. Treat for shock if not resolved with repositioning.

H. Pulmonary embolism

1. Can occur anytime during or shortly after pregnancy.

2. Signs and symptoms

    i. Acute onset dyspnea

    ii. Chest pain

3. Management

    i. Provide general management of ALS patients.

    ii. Rapid transport

I. Maternal cardiac arrest

1. Attempt to determine gestational age.

2. Begin CPR per current AHA BLS guidelines.

Note: Do *not* use mechanical CPR devices for maternal cardiac arrest patients.

3. Manually displace uterus off aorta and vena cava (left uterine displacement).

    i. Effective chest compression can be generated with patients inclined at angles of up to 30°. Any cushion or pillow can be used to wedge the patient into the left inclined position. Manually move the uterus further off the inferior vena cava by lifting it with two hands to the left and towards the patient's head.

4. Defibrillate VF and PVT per current AHA ACLS guidelines.

5. Provide rapid airway management and ventilation with 100% oxygen. (*No* hyperventilation.)

6. Administer emergency drugs per current AHA ACLS guidelines.

7. Transport to appropriate hospital with perimortem Caesarean capability.

V. STAGES OF LABOR

A. Stage one—from onset of true labor through full cervical dilation

B. Stage two—from full cervical dilation through delivery of the newborn

C. Stage three—from delivery of newborn through delivery of the placenta

D. Stage four—recovery of the mother

VI. NORMAL FIELD DELIVERY

A. Prepare OB kit.

B. Position mother (not supine).

C. Assess for crowning.

D. If necessary, manually rupture amniotic sac to facilitate delivery.

E. Assess for presence of thick meconium in amniotic fluid.

F. Support head, guide external rotation (avoid fontanelles).

G. Ensure cord is not around baby's neck.

H. Guide, presenting should be up, then guide down to facilitate delivery.

I. Begin newborn assessment and interventions as indicated.

J. Clamp and cut cord once done pulsating.

K. Make transport decision while awaiting placental delivery.

L. Prepare for delivery of placenta. Gently guide, do not pull.

M. Monitor postpartum hemorrhage, signs of shock.

N. Uterine massage and/or breastfeeding can reduce postpartum hemorrhage.

O. Transport mother, baby, and placenta.

 VII. **NEWBORN CARE/NEONATAL RESUSCITATION**—See Chapter 24

 VIII. **ABNORMAL DELIVERY COMPLICATIONS**

A. Breech presentation

   1. Either both feet or buttocks present first in birth canal.

   2. Management

      i. Transport rapidly if possible for possible Caesarean.

      ii. Support baby during delivery.

      iii. If head becomes trapped, form a "V" with fingers in birth canal over baby's face to facilitate breathing.

B. Prolapsed cord

   1. Umbilical cord is presenting partly, before the baby.

   2. Cord can become compressed during delivery, shutting down fetal circulation.

   3. Management

      i.   Do *not* attempt delivery.

      ii. Use gloved hand to gently ease fetus off the cord.

      iii. Place mother in knee-chest position.

      iv. Transport immediately to appropriate facility.

C. Limb presentation

   1. Arm or leg is presenting part.

   2. Do *not* attempt delivery.

   3. Place mother in knee-chest position.

   4. Cover limb to prevent heat loss.

   5. Transport immediately for Caesarean.

D. Nuchal cord

   1. Cord is wrapped around baby's neck.

   2. Management

      i.   Gently slip cord over baby's head. (This usually works.)

      ii. If cord compression occurs and unable to slip cord over baby's head—clamp the cord in two places (2" apart) and cut.

> ***Note:*** Determine possibility of multiple births before making decision to cut umbilical cord.

E. Multiple births

   1. Have increased risk of preterm labor and low birth weight hypothermia.

   2. You need to request additional resources and prepare additional equipment.

   3. May be one shared or two separate placentas.

F. Meconium

1. Is the presence of fetal stool in amniotic fluid.

2. Appears as thick light yellow to green "pea soup" colored amniotic fluid.

3. Indicates likelihood of fetal hypoxia.

4. Increased risk of aspiration and infection.

5. Management

   i. No intervention needed for light meconium staining.

   ii. For thick meconium, suction airway as able to reduce aspiration risk.

   iii. Consider use of endotracheal tube and meconium aspirator attached to suction.

IX. GYNECOLOGICAL EMERGENCIES

A. Ectopic pregnancy

1. Pregnancy where the fertilized egg implants outside of the uterus, usually in the fallopian tubes.

2. A ruptured fallopian tube will cause massive hemorrhage.

3. Requires rapid surgical intervention.

4. Signs and symptoms

   i. Diffuse abdominal tenderness progressing to sharp, localized, unilateral lower quadrant abdominal pain (may radiate to shoulder).

   ii. Late or missed menstrual cycle

   iii. Vaginal bleeding

   iv. Signs and symptoms of shock

> *Note:* Encourage transport for any female patient of childbearing years with abdominal pain for suspected ectopic pregnancy.

B. Pelvic Inflammatory Disease (PID)

1. Infection of female reproductive tract, including gonorrhea and chlamydia.

2. Can be acute or chronic and lead to infertility, ectopic pregnancy, and sepsis.

3. Signs and symptoms

   i. Diffuse lower abdominal pain

   ii. Increased pain with intercourse or walking

   iii. Fever, chills

   iv. N&V

   v. Foul-smelling vaginal discharge

   vi. Mid-cycle vaginal bleeding

C. Ovarian cyst

1. Fluid-filled pockets in the ovary that can rupture.

2. Signs and symptoms

   i. Severe unilateral abdominal pain

   ii. Vaginal bleeding

D. Endometriosis

1. Disorder causing uterine tissue to develop outside of the uterus.

2. Signs and symptoms

   i. Dull, cramping pelvic or lower abdominal pain

   ii. Abnormal menstrual bleeding

E. Sexual assault

1. Victims of sexual assault can be male or female, young or old. Patients are often females with possible gynecologic trauma.

2. First priority is patient care, then reporting to appropriate authorities, e.g., law enforcement, or child or adult protective services.

3. Guidelines for management of sexual assault victims:

    i.   Treat patient first, preserve evidence second.

    ii.   Provide psychological support.

    iii. Provide same-sex EMS provider when possible.

    iv. Do not disrupt possible crime scene any more than necessary.

    v.   Handle clothing as little as possible.

    vi. Place any clothing or bloody items that have been removed in brown paper bags.

    vii. Do not cut through tears or holes in clothing.

    viii. Only examine perineal area if necessary to manage significant injury.

    ix. Encourage patient not to change clothes, urinate, shower, or douche prior to medical examination at hospital.

F. General management of gynecological patients

1. Provide general management of ALS patients.

2. Treat for shock as indicated.

3. Remember, females of childbearing years with abdominal pain should be treated and transported for possible ectopic pregnancy until ruled out.

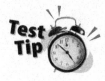

You will not likely see many questions with "all of the above" or "none of the above" answer choices. This is good! Use caution with any questions that include the word "except." Unlike most questions, "except" questions usually have three correct answer choices and one incorrect choice. You are looking for the incorrect choice. Slow down and read these questions carefully.

Neonatology

> **Note:** For information about general management of ALS patients, see Chapter 4.

I. TERMS TO KNOW

A. Acrocyanosis—cyanosis of the hands and feet due to poor perfusion

B. Gestation—time from conception to birth

C. Meconium—fecal material in amniotic fluid from baby's first bowel movement

D. Neonate—newborns from birth to one-month old

E. Patent ductus arteriosus—ductus arteriosus fails to close during embryonic development causing aortic blood flow into pulmonary artery

F. Preterm—infant delivered prior to 37 weeks gestation

II. PATHOPHYSIOLOGY

A. Risk factors for newborn complications

1. Multiple gestation pregnancies

2. No prenatal care

3. Mother under 16 or over 35 years of age

4. Drug or alcohol abuse during pregnancy

5. Preterm labor

6. Meconium

7. Amniotic sac ruptures more than 24 hours prior to delivery

8. Abnormal presentation during delivery

9. Prolonged labor or explosive delivery

B. Resuscitation

1. About 10% of newborns require assistance to begin breathing.

2. About 1% require full resuscitative measures.

3. Need for resuscitation inversely related to birth weight (about 80% of newborns under 3.5 lbs. require resuscitation).

4. Cardiac arrest in neonates usually due to hypoxia.

III. CONGENITAL ANOMALIES

A. A leading cause of death among infants.

B. Congenital heart defects

1. May increase pulmonary flow causing CHF.

2. May decrease pulmonary flow compromising oxygenation.

3. May obstruct blood flow.

C. Diaphragmatic hernia

1. Abdominal contents enter thorax through opening in diaphragm (rare).

2. Signs and symptoms

i. Dyspnea and cyanosis unresponsive to oxygenation and ventilation

ii. Bowel sounds auscultated in the chest

iii. Flat abdomen

3. Management

    i.   Position head and thorax above abdomen.

    ii. Insert OG or NG tube with low, intermittent suction (facilitates improved ventilation).

    iii. Do *not* initiate BVM ventilation without intubation (increases gastric distention). Intubate if BVM ventilations are necessary.

    iv. Employ rapid transport for surgical repair.

D. Spina bifida

1. Spinal cord is exposed. Cover with moist, sterile, occlusive dressing, and place newborn in prone or lateral position.

IV. NEWBORN ASSESSMENT AND RESUSCITATION

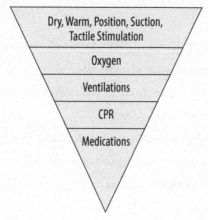

Inverted Pyramid of Neonatal Resuscitation

Dry, Warm, Position, Suction, Tactile Stimulation

Oxygen

Ventilations

CPR

Medications

A. Routine delivery (term newborn, good muscle tone, breathing adequately)

1. Routine care: keep warm and dry, clear secretions as indicated.

2. Normal Assessment Findings in Newborns

Normal Vitals	Normal Blood Glucose
➤ Respirations: 40–60/min	➤ At least 45 mg/dL
➤ Pulse: 100–180/min	**Normal Weight**
Normal SpO$_2$	➤ About 5½–8½ lbs
➤ At least 93%	**Normal APGAR**
Normal Temp	➤ 7–10
➤ 98–100 degrees F (36.7–37.8 C)	

B. *Not* routine delivery (not term, underweight, poor muscle tone, not breathing adequately)

> ***Note:*** Refer to current AHA Neonatal Resuscitation Algorithm, available online.

1. Dry, warm, position, suction, tactile stimulation

2. Check respirations and heart rate

   i.   If breathing adequately and heart rate over 100.

      ➤ Check skin color.

      ➤ Monitor SpO$_2$, administer blow-by oxygen as indicated.

3. If apneic/gasping breaths or heart rate below 100

   i.   Begin BVM ventilations.

   ii. Monitor SpO$_2$/ECG monitoring.

> ***Note:*** All of the above interventions should not take longer than one minute.

4. Check heart rate

   i.   If heart rate over 100, provide supportive care.

   ii. Heart rate below 100

      ➤ Ensure adequate PPV and recheck heart rate.

➤ Heart rate below 60

— Intubate.

— Begin CPR (3:1 compressions: ventilations).

— Ensure adequate BVM with 100% oxygen.

— Reassess heart rate.

— If below 60, IV epinephrine, assess for hypovolemia, pneumothorax.

➤ Heart rate over 60, below 100

— Continue BVM ventilation with 100% O_2.

➤ Heart rate over 100

— Supportive care

B. APGAR scoring

1. Assess APGAR at 1 minute and 5 minutes post-delivery.

APGAR Scoring (0–10)		
Appearance (skin)	Pink (everywhere)	2
	Pink (core only)	1
	Cyanosis (central)	0
Pulse (rate)	Over 100/min	2
	Under 100	1
	Absent	0
Grimace (irritability)	Crying	2
	Grimacing	1
	No response	0
Activity (muscle tone)	Active	2
	Some motion	1
	Limp	0
Respirations (effort)	Strong cry	2
	Slow or irregular	1
	Absent	0
7–10: likely only routine care needed 4–6: likely stimulation/oxygenation needed 0–3: Begin resuscitation immediately.		

Note: Do **not** delay critical interventions for newborns to obtain an APGAR score.

C. Special considerations

    i.   Bulb syringe—Routine suctioning with bulb syringe *no longer recommended* (can stimulate the vagus nerve, causing bradycardia and hypoxia).

    ii.   Suction—If amniotic fluid is clear, do not suction unless airway is obstructed or BVM is required.

1. Meconium

    i.   For thick meconium in nonvigorous newborns, quickly clear airway and initiate ventilations within one minute of delivery (before stimulating to breathe).

    ii.   Use endotracheal tube (ETT) connected to meconium aspirator to suction trachea (100 cm/H_2O of suction or less).

    iii.   Do not intubate with contaminated ETT, use a new one.

    iv.   Quickly oxygenate and ventilate as indicated.

Note: Suctioning can increase hypoxia and should be completed quickly.

2. Gastric decompression (OG/NG tube) indicated for newborns with gastric distention (often due to prolonged BVM ventilation).

3. Medications administration

    i.   Consider umbilical vein and IO for vascular access for medications.

    ii.   Epinephrine administration per current ACLS guidelines

    iii.   Naloxone *no longer indicated* in newborn resuscitation, as it can cause withdrawal syndrome

    iv.   If IV fluids indicated, administer 10 mL/kg of normal saline or lactated Ringers.

    v.   If dextrose indicated for hypoglycemia (below 45 mg/dL), use 10% dextrose solution (D10, NOT D50).

D. Cutting the cord

1. There is no urgency to clamp and cut the cord *unless* resuscitation measures are needed.

2. Delayed cord clamping acceptable for vigorous newborns who are adequately breathing and crying.

3. Place one clamp about 4″ from newborn and another clamp 2″ further and cut between clamps.

 V. NEONATAL EMERGENCIES

A. Bradycardia

1. The primary cause of bradycardia in pediatric patients (including newborns) is hypoxia.

2. *Always* manage a bradycardic newborn/infant/pediatric patient for hypoxia first, then consider other causes, e.g., increased ICP, cardiac anomalies, metabolic problem, medications, etc.

3. Remember to begin CPR for any unresponsive pediatric patient with a pulse below 60 beats per minute.

B. Premature newborn

1. Newborn delivered prior to 37 weeks gestation

2. Increased risk of

   i. Underweight newborn (under about 5.5 lbs)

   ii. Respiratory compromise

   iii. Hypothermia

   iv. Head bleeds

3. Management

   i. Treat as regular newborn.

   ii. Resuscitate as indicated per AHA guidelines.

   iii. Manage hypoxia and hypothermia as indicated.

   iv. Rapid transport to appropriate facility.

C. Hypovolemia

1. Leading cause of shock in newborns

   i. Dehydration (diarrhea, vomiting, fever) most common cause

   ii. Hemorrhage

   iii. Third spacing of fluids

2. Signs and symptoms

   i. Pale, cool skin

   ii. Weak or absent peripheral pulses

   iii. Delayed capillary refill (not associated with hypothermia)

   iv. Decreased LOC

   v. Decreased urinary output (dark urine or dry diaper)

3. Management

   i. IV/IO fluids (NS or LR) at 10 mL/kg over 5–10 minutes and reassess

   ii. Repeat as indicated (40–60 mL/kg may be needed).

D. Seizures

1. Generalized tonic-clonic seizures rare in neonates. Instead they are usually:

   i. Subtle seizures with apnea and swim or pedal-like movements.

   ii. Tonic (rigid) seizures.

   iii. Focal clonic seizures.

   iv. Myoclonic seizures (brief focal or generalized jerking of extremities).

2. Common causes of neonatal seizures

   i. Seizures in newborns suggestive of neurological disorder

   ii. Hypoglycemia (blood glucose below 45 mg/dL)

   iii. Sepsis

   iv. Fever

   v. Meningitis

   vi. Medication withdrawal

3. Management

   i.   Conduct general management of ALS patients.

   ii.   Anticonvulsant meds per local protocol

   iii.   Dextrose (D10) for hypoglycemia

   iv.   Employ rapid transport.

E. Fever

1. Normal newborn temp: 99.5 degrees F (37.5C)

2. Rectal temp of 100.4 degrees F (38C) is considered febrile.

   i.   Oral temp about 1 degree F below rectal

   ii.   Axillary temp about 2 degrees F below rectal

3. Any neonate with a fever should be treated for possible sepsis or meningitis.

4. Do *not* apply cold packs.

5. Transport.

F. Neonatal jaundice

1. Is usually due to excess bilirubin caused by liver immaturity.

2. Can last one to two weeks after delivery.

3. Is usually treated successfully with phototherapy (light).

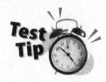

The test will end for one of three reasons:

1. **The test ends because you passed (you!) or failed (not you!).**

2. **The test ends because time is up. Over 99% of candidates finish the exam in the time allowed.**

3. **The test ends because you reached the maximum number of questions. Paramedic candidates will see between 80–150 questions.**

Pediatrics

Note: For information about general management of ALS patients, see Chapter 4.

I. TERMS TO KNOW

A. Intussusception—telescoping of intestines into themselves. Usually occurs in patients 6 months to 6 years. Requires surgery.

B. Mottling—abnormal skin coloring due to vasoconstriction and poor circulation

C. Neglect—failure of caregiver to provide basic necessities

D. Petechiae—small, purple, non-blanching spots on skin

E. Respiratory arrest—apnea

F. Respiratory distress—increased rate and effort of breathing

G. Respiratory failure—inadequate oxygenation and ventilation

H. Tenting—poor skin turgor (slow retraction of skin after being pinched), indicating possible dehydration

II. NORMAL VITALS AND PEDIATRIC DEVELOPMENTAL CHARACTERISTICS

A. Neonates (up to one month)

1. Normal heart rate: 100–180

2. Normal respiratory rate: 30–60

3. Normal systolic BP: at least 60

B. Infants (1 month–1 year)

1. Normal heart rate: 100–160

2. Normal respiratory rate: 30–60

3. Normal systolic BP: at least 70

C. Toddlers (1–3 years)

1. Normal heart rate: 80–110

2. Normal respiratory rate: 24–40

3. Minimal acceptable systolic BP: at least 70 + 2(age)

D. Preschoolers (3–5 years)

1. Normal heart rate: 70–110

2. Normal respiratory rate: 22–34

3. Minimal acceptable systolic BP: at least 70 + 2(age)

E. School age (6–12 years)

1. Normal heart rate: 65–110

2. Normal respiratory rate: 18–30

3. Minimal acceptable systolic BP: at least 70 + 2(age)

F. Adolescents (13–18 years)

1. Normal heart rate: 60–90

2. Normal respiratory rate: 12–26

3. Normal systolic BP: approaching adult values

Pediatric Developmental Characteristics

	Physical Development	Cognitive Development
Birth to 6 months	• Turns head/controls gaze • Recognizes caregivers (2–6 months) • Makes eye contact (2–6 months) • Rolls over (2–6 months)	• Communicates by crying • Trust develops • Increased awareness of surroundings (2–6 months) • Seeks attention (2–6 months)
6 to 12 months	• Can sit/crawl • Puts anything in mouth • Teething	• Babbles • Object curiosity • Separation anxiety/tantrums
12 to 18 months	• Crawls/walks • Sensory development	• Imitates • Understands "make believe" • Begins developing vocabulary • Separation anxiety
18 to 24 months	• Runs/climbs • Good balance	• Understands cause/effect • Vocabulary improves • Object attachment
Preschool	• Physically active	• Highly verbal and literal • Can set goals • Monster fear • Can feel guilt
School Age	• Approaching adult anatomy • Breast development/ onset of menstrual cycle in females	• Analytical • Peer/popularity concerns

III. ANATOMY AND PHYSIOLOGY REVIEW

A. Head

  1. Infant fontanelles may take up to 18 months to completely close.

    i. Bulging fontanelle may indicate increased ICP.

    ii. Sunken fontanelle may indicate hypovolemia.

2. Pediatric head is proportionally larger than an adult's.

    i.   Increased risk of head injury

    ii.   Difficult to maintain mask seal during BVM ventilation

B. Airway

1. Pediatric tongue proportionally larger (Airway can obstruct more easily.)

2. Airway management

    i.   Do *not* hyperextend head (can close off airway).

    ii.   Under 3 years: pad behind shoulders to place airway in neutral position.

    iii. Over 3 years: may need to pad behind occiput to obtain sniffing position.

    iv. Cricoid ring (below cords) narrowest part of younger pediatric airways.

    v.   Infants are obligate nose breathers (easily causes respiratory compromise).

C. Chest & Lungs

1. Pediatric patients are often abdominal breathers.

2. Higher metabolic rate

    i.   Greater oxygen demand

    ii.   Higher resting respiratory rates

    iii. Lower oxygen reserves and increased risk of hypoxia

3. Pliable ribs increase risk of injury to underlying organs, e.g., pulmonary contusion, pneumothorax.

D. Cardiovascular

1. Limited cardiovascular reserves

2. Higher resting heart rate

E. Shock

　1. Maintain blood pressure longer, despite significant shock.

　2. Hypotension is a very LATE sign of shock.

　3. Normal presence of tachycardia can mask shock.

IV. PEDIATRIC ASSESSMENT TRIANGLE (PAT)

A. Used to quickly inform general impression: sick or not sick/hurt or not hurt.

B. Intended to be a visual and auditory assessment that can be completed before stressing a child with a hands-on assessment.

C. An abnormal finding in any of the three components of PAT can indicate need for rapid stabilization and rapid transport.

D. The ABCs of the PAT

　1. *Appearance* (mental status and muscle tone)

　　i.　Tone

　　ii.　Interactivity

　　iii.　Consolability

　　iv.　Look/gaze

　　v.　Speech/cry

> **Note:** Abnormalities here may indicate CNS problem, e.g., altered LOC, seizures, toxicology, diabetic problem, etc.

　2. Work of *Breathing* (respiratory rate and effort)

　　i.　Accessory muscle use/retractions/flaring

　　ii.　Abnormal airway sounds

　　iii.　Posturing/tripod breathing

　　iv.　After PAT: auscultate lung sounds

> ***Note:*** Abnormalities here may indicate respiratory problem (trauma or medical).

3. *Circulation* to skin (skin color)
   i. Skin color (normal, pale, mottled, cyanotic)
   ii. After PAT
       ➤ Capillary refill
       ➤ Central v. peripheral pulses
       ➤ Temperature

> ***Note:*** Abnormalities here may indicate shock (trauma or medical).

E. Use PAT to help determine transport priority.
   1. Urgent: manage immediate life threats (primary and rapid secondary) and transport immediately.
   2. Nonurgent: can complete secondary assessment on scene prior to transport.

V. PEDIATRIC ASSESSMENT TIPS

A. Tachypnea is an early sign of respiratory distress.

B. A slowing respiratory rate may indicate impending respiratory failure.

C. Nasal flaring is a sign of respiratory distress.

D. Cyanosis in mucous membranes and nail beds is a late sign of respiratory failure.

E. Cyanosis of the extremities only indicates shock.

F. Capillary refill is a reliable sign of perfusion only in patients under 6 years of age.

> *Note:* Capillary refill over 2 seconds indicates poor perfusion.

G. Maintain high index of suspicion for dehydration (vomiting, diarrhea, dry diapers, skin tending, poor circulation etc.).

H. Altered LOC may indicate poor CNS perfusion, e.g., inconsolable or unable to recognize parents.

I. Bradycardia, especially in a distressed infant or pediatric patient, likely indicates impending cardiac arrest.

J. Strong peripheral pulses indicate adequate perfusion.

K. Decreased peripheral perfusion is an early indication of shock.

VI. RISK FACTORS FOR IMPENDING CARDIAC ARREST

A. Respirations over 60 per minute

B. Pulse rate under 80 or over 180 (patients under 5 years of age)

C. Respiratory distress

D. Trauma or burn injuries

E. Cyanosis

F. ALOC

G. Seizures

H. Fever with petechiae

> *Note:* Cardiac arrest in pediatric patients is usually caused by respiratory failure or shock.

VII. PEDIATRIC MANAGEMENT TIPS

A. Basic airway management

1. Use OPAs only for unresponsive patients without gag reflex.

2. Insert with use of a tongue blade.

3. Do *not* insert OPA with 180-degree rotation as with adults.

4. Do *not* use NPAs on patients with suspected face or head trauma.

5. Size OPAs and NPAs as with adults.

6. Decrease suction pressure (max 100 mmHg in infants).

7. Decrease suction time to reduce hypoxia.

B. Advanced airway management

1. Calculating pediatric endotracheal tube (ETT) size: (16 + age in years) ÷ 4

2. Verify proper ETT placement: see Chapter 3.

> **Note:** Use resuscitation tape, app, or card for appropriate tube size, depth, etc.

C. Ventilation

1. Avoid hyperventilation during BVM ventilation.

2. Utilize waveform capnography when available.

3. Do *not* use flow-restricted, oxygen-powered ventilatory device on pediatric patients.

4. Avoid BVM devices with pop-off valves.

5. Insert OG or NG tube as indicated for gastric decompression.

SPECIFIC PEDIATRIC EMERGENCIES

A. See previous chapters for the following:

1. Asthma: see Chapter 8

2. Croup: see Chapter 3

3. Drowning: see Chapter 22

4. Diabetes: see Chapter 10

5. Meningitis: see Chapter 14

6. Pneumonia: see Chapter 8

7. Poisoning/OD: see Chapter 13

8. Seizures: see Chapter 9

B. Bronchopulmonary dysplasia

1. Is a chronic lung disease that typically affects premature newborns and infants.

2. Bronchi and alveoli are damaged in the neonatal period, often due to PPV and high-concentration oxygen.

3. Causes recurrent respiratory infections and exercised-induced bronchospasm.

4. Management may include inhaled bronchodilators, CPAP, and PPV as indicated.

C. Epiglottitis

1. Is an acute infection/inflammation of the epiglottis.

2. Is rare, but potentially life-threatening due to airway obstruction.

3. Signs and symptoms

   i. Acute onset fever and cough

   ii. Sore throat

   iii. Dyspnea

   iv. Stridor

   v. Drooling

      vi.   Tripod breathing

      vii. Accessory muscle use

  4. Management

     i.   Do *not* aggravate child (may worsen airway compromise).

       ➤ Do *not* visualize airway, force suction, start prophylactic IV, etc.

     ii.   Use supplemental oxygen as tolerated by patient (humidified when possible).

     iii. Consider nebulized bronchodilators per local protocol.

     iv. Initiate BVM ventilation as indicated (avoid intubation when able).

D. Bronchiolitis

  1. Respiratory infection of the bronchioles

  2. Typically occurs in winter, children under 2 years of age.

  3. Signs and symptoms:

     i.   Similar to asthma

     ii.   Expiratory wheezing

  4. Management

     i.   Conduct general management of ALS patients.

     ii.   Place in position of comfort.

     iii. Use nebulized bronchodilators per local protocol.

E. Sudden infant death syndrome (SIDS)

  1. Sudden death of infant from unknown etiology.

  2. A leading cause of death in infants (especially 1–6 months old).

  3. Management

     i.   Follow normal resuscitation guidelines.

     ii.   Support parents/family members.

     iii. If resuscitation is not initiated or terminated, allow family to see child.

F. Apparent life-threatening event (ALTE)

    1. Sudden occurrence of certain symptoms

        i. Apnea

        ii. Cyanosis

        iii. Loss of muscle tone

        iv. Coughing or gagging

    2. Transport patients if history indicates occurrence of ALTE.

G. Abuse or neglect

    1. Perpetrators

        i. Are usually a parent or full-time caregiver.

        ii. Often exhibit evasive or hostile behavior.

        iii. May be experiencing crisis, financial stress, relationship issues.

    2. Types of abuse

        i. Psychological abuse

        ii. Physical abuse

        iii. Sexual abuse

        iv. Neglect

    3. Signs and symptoms

        i. Unexplained injuries, fractures, burns, TBI

        ii. Multiple injuries in various stages of healing

        iii. Injuries over multiple areas of body

        iv. History that doesn't match MOI

        v. Delay in seeking medical attention

        vi. Malnutrition

        vii. Skin infections

        viii. Poor hygiene

        ix. Delayed verbal or social skills

4. Management

    i.   Provide proper medical attention.

    ii.   Do everything possible to facilitate transport.

    iii.   Report suspicions to authorities.

    iv.   Document thoroughly.

H. Patients with special needs

1. Tracheostomy tube: see Chapter 3.

2. Home ventilator

    i.   9-1-1 calls often due to mechanical failure or loss of electricity.

    ii.   Switch immediately to BVM ventilation until problem resolved and transport as indicated.

3. Central line

    i.   Used for long-term IV therapies.

    ii.   Includes percutaneous intravenous catheters (PIC) lines.

    iii.   Complications

        ➤ Obstruction of line (clotting, cracked or kinked line)

        ➤ Site infection

        ➤ Hemorrhage

        ➤ Air embolism

    iv.   Management

        ➤ Control bleeding.

        ➤ Clamp line if large amount of air in line.

        ➤ Place patient on left side with head down if air embolism suspected.

        ➤ Transport.

4. Gastric tube

    i.   Gastric tubes (inserted nasally into stomach) and gastronomy tubes (placed through abdominal wall into stomach) used for patients not capable of eating normally

    ii.   Complications

        ➤ Bleeding

        ➤ Displaced tube

    iii. Management

       ➤ Supportive care

       ➤ Minimize risk of aspiration

       ➤ Transport

5. Shunt

    i. Surgical procedure allowing excess CSF to drain from brain to abdomen, reducing risk of increased ICP

    ii. Signs of shunt failure

       ➤ Altered LOC

       ➤ Posturing

       ➤ Pupillary changes

    iii. Management

       ➤ General management of ALS patients

       ➤ Rapid transport for surgical intervention

IX. JUMPSTART TRIAGE (MASS CASUALTY INCIDENTS)

A. Based on START triage (see Chapter 29)

1. GREEN = Minor patients

2. YELLOW = Delayed patients

3. RED = Immediate patients

4. BLACK = Expectant (dead/dying) patients

B. If patient appears to be a child, use JumpSTART algorithm

1. Don't delay triage to confirm age.

2. See JumpSTART algorithm.

C. JumpSTART special considerations.

1. Triage patients too young to walk and nonambulatory patients (as these patients cannot move themselves to GREEN (Minor) area).

2. Once RED (immediate) patients and YELLOW (delayed) patients are managed, reassess BLACK (expectant) patients.

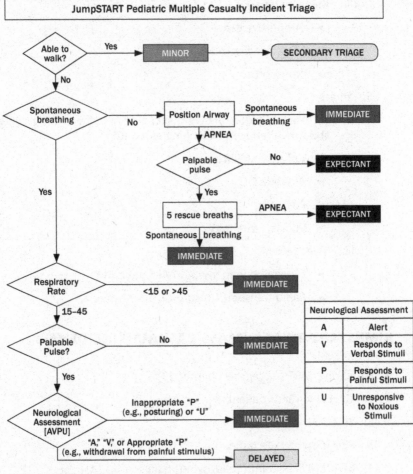

JumpSTART Pediatric Multiple Casualty Incident Triage

Able to walk? — Yes → MINOR → SECONDARY TRIAGE

No

Spontaneous breathing — No → Position Airway — Spontaneous breathing → IMMEDIATE

APNEA

Palpable pulse — No → EXPECTANT

Yes

5 rescue breaths — APNEA → EXPECTANT

Spontaneous breathing → IMMEDIATE

Yes

Respiratory Rate — <15 or >45 → IMMEDIATE

15–45

Palpable Pulse? — No → IMMEDIATE

Yes

Neurological Assessment [AVPU] — Inappropriate "P" (e.g., posturing) or "U" → IMMEDIATE

"A," "V," or Appropriate "P" (e.g., withdrawal from painful stimulus) → DELAYED

Neurological Assessment	
A	Alert
V	Responds to Verbal Stimuli
P	Responds to Painful Stimuli
U	Unresponsive to Noxious Stimuli

Use JumpSTART if the Patient appears to be a child.
Use an adult system, such as START, if the patient appears to be a young adult.

Triage Categories

EXPECTANT Black Triage Tag Color

- Victim unlikely to survive given severity of injuries, level of available care, or both
- Palliative care and pain relief should be provided

IMMEDIATE Red Triage Tag Color

- Victim can be helped by immediate intervention and transport
- Requires medical attention within minutes for survival (up to 60)
- Includes compromises to patient's Airway, Breathing, Circulation

DELAYED Yellow Triage Tag Color

- Victim's transport can be delayed
- Includes serious and potentially life-threatening injuries, but status not expected to deteriorate significantly over several hours

MINOR Green Triage Tag Color

- Victim with relatively minor injuries
- Status unlikely to deteriorate over days
- May be able to assist in own care: "Walking Wounded"

X. CHILD PASSENGER SAFETY

A. Birth–2 years: rear-facing seat, back seat

B. 2–5 years: forward-facing seat, back seat

C. 5+ years: seatbelts fit properly: booster seat. Belts fit properly when the lap belt lays across the upper thighs (not stomach) and the shoulder belt lays across the chest (not neck). Back seat for the best protection.

> **Note:** Buckle all children 12 and under in back seat (middle seat preferred). Never place rear-facing seat in front of an airbag.

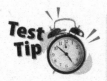

> *The national certification exam is based on the two current American Heart Association guidelines: Basic Life Support (BLS) and Advanced Cardiovascular Life Support (ACLS). If you are unsure about your knowledge of these guidelines, review the appropriate AHA textbook or equivalent publications.*

Geriatrics

I. TERMS TO KNOW

A. Functional impairment—loss of ability to independently meet daily needs

B. Geriatric—someone who is at least 65 years of age

C. Gerontology—the study of the effects of aging on humans

D. Incontinence—accidental urination or defecation

E. Polypharmacy—concurrent use of multiple medications

F. Proprioception—ability to perceive or sense movements and position of one's own body, independent of vision

II. PATHOPHYSIOLOGY OF AGING

A. Multi-system deterioration

1. Physical maintenance, immune defense, and injury repair processes slow and weaken with age.

2. Most elderly patients have multiple medical conditions simultaneously.

B. Common chief complaints

1. Weakness

2. Dizziness, syncope

3. Falls

4. Headache

5. Insomnia

6. Loss of appetite

7. GI/GU problems

C. Pharmacology

1. Most elderly patients take at least four different prescription medications.

2. Patients taking at least six different medications have a high risk of dangerous medication interaction.

3. Large percentage of elderly patients does not take meds as prescribed (noncompliance).

4. Beta blockers

    i.   Commonly prescribed to elderly for hypertension, angina, cardiac dysrhythmias

    ii. Side effects often poorly tolerated in elderly

         ➤ Lethargy

         ➤ Depression

         ➤ Dizziness

         ➤ GI problems

    iii. Commonly prescribed beta blockers

         ➤ Propranolol (Inderal)

         ➤ Atenolol

         ➤ Metoprolol

         ➤ Labetalol

5. Angiotensin-converting enzyme (ACE) inhibitors

    i.   Used for hypertension and CHF

    ii. Commonly prescribed ACE inhibitors

         ➤ Captopril

         ➤ Lisinopril

         ➤ Benazepril

iii. Side effects

> ➤ Hypotension

> ➤ Vomiting

> ➤ Diarrhea

6. Digitalis (Digoxin, Lanoxin)

   i. Widely prescribed for CHF and cardiac dysrhythmias

   ii. Has positive inotropic and negative chronotropic effects

   iii. High risk of toxicity, presenting with:

   > ➤ Visual disturbances

   > ➤ Weakness, fatigue

   > ➤ Nausea & vomiting (N&V)

   > ➤ Headache

D. Falls

1. Elderly have a higher risk of falls than most other age groups and a higher risk of death due to fall-related injuries.

III. GERIATRIC "GEMS" ASSESSMENT

A. Geriatric patients

1. Remember, geriatrics have atypical presentations for various conditions.

B. Environmental assessment

1. Check safety, cleanliness of patient's living environment.

2. Working plumbing, heating, cooling, etc.?

3. Signs of alcohol abuse?

4. Fall risks?

5. Access to phone?

6. Prescribed medications present and not expired?

C. **M**edical assessment

    1. Expect multiple medical problems and medications.

    2. Does trauma indicate a preceding medical condition?

    3. Signs of abuse, neglect, malnutrition, dehydration, etc.

D. **S**ocial assessment

    1. Assess activities of daily living (eating, dressing, bathing, etc.).

    2. Any difficulties obtaining food, medications, etc.

    3. Family support? Social network?

IV. COMMON MEDICAL CONDITIONS IN THE ELDERLY

A. Pneumonia (Chapter 14)

    1. Elderly pneumonia patient may not present with fever.

B. Myocardial infarction

    1. Risk of angina, MI increases with age.

    2. Mortality rate doubles after age 70.

    3. Elderly more likely to present atypical MI symptoms

        i.   Lack of chest pain

        ii. Indigestion, epigastric pain

        iii. Dizziness, syncope

        iv. Dyspnea

        v. Fatigue

C. Congestive heart failure (Chapter 7)

    1. One of the most common causes of hospitalization after age 60.

    2. AMI is a common cause of heart failure.

D. Hypertension

    1. About half of all elderly patients have some degree of hypertension.

2. Signs may be subtle in elderly.

    i.   Headache

    ii. Tinnitus

    iii. Epistaxis

    iv. May indicate thyroid disease

E. Syncope

  1. One of the most common chief complaints

  2. Indicates need for thorough ALS-level assessment.

  3. Always question patients who have fallen about possible syncopal episode.

F. Stroke

  1. There is an increased risk of stroke and TIA in elderly.

  2. One-third of those with TIAs will have a stroke.

G. Seizures

  1. Common causes in elderly

    i.   Alcohol withdrawal

    ii. Hypoglycemia

    iii. Tumor or cerebral hemorrhage

    iv. TBI

    v. Epilepsy

    vi. Stroke

  2. Common antiseizure meds

    i.   Tegretol

    ii. Zarontin

    iii. Neurontin

    iv. Keppra

    v. Luminal

    vi. Dilantin

      vii. Depakote

     viii. Depakene

H. Delirium, dementia, Alzheimer's

  1. Delirium

      i. An acute change in mentation

      ii. Many serious causes, some reversible

     iii. Affects mentation more than memory.

     iv. Indicates need for high priority transport.

  2. Dementia

      i. Slow, progressive, and often irreversible deterioration in mentation

      ii. Affects memory more than mentation.

     iii. Usually caused by Alzheimer's disease.

     iv. Does not usually require high priority transport.

  3. Alzheimer's disease

      i. A form of dementia

      ii. Signs and symptoms

         ➤ Loss of recent memories

         ➤ Difficulty learning new things

         ➤ Mood swings, personality changes

         ➤ Wandering, often at night

         ➤ Functional impairment

         ➤ Frequent falls

         ➤ Regression to infant stage

I. Parkinson's disease

  1. Degenerative disorder

  2. Signs and symptoms

      i. Tremors

      ii. Ambulatory difficulties, shuffling gait

       iii.   Loss of facial expression

       iv.   Muscle rigidity

       v.   Jerky motion

       vi.   Slow, monotone speech

J. Suicide (Chapter 15)

   1. Highest suicide rates are in patients (especially males) over 65.

K. Trauma and falls

   1. Increased risk of injury and death, even from ground-level falls

   2. Risk factors

       i.   Poor health

       ii.   Polypharmacy, use of blood thinners, beta blockers

       iii.   Increased risk of abuse, neglect

       iv.   Living in home environment without fall prevention measures

   3. Most common fall-related fractures are to hip or pelvis, increasing risk of death.

   4. Assume elderly fall victim has a hip or pelvic fracture until proven otherwise.

L. Elder abuse, neglect

   1. Can occur domestically (at home) or institutionally (in a care center).

   2. Risk factors

       i.   Loss of independence

       ii.   Living in nursing home or care facility or cared for by family member under great stress

   3. Signs of abuse or neglect

       i.   See Chapter 25

       ii.   Signs of malnutrition

       iii.   Bed sores/pressure sores

       iv.   Poor hygiene or living conditions

4. Suspected abuse or neglect must be reported to appropriate authorities, as with suspected child abuse.

M. Herpes zoster

1. Also known as shingles.

2. Causes painful rash with blisters. Pain can continue after rash resolves.

3. Risk increases with age.

4. Chickenpox vaccine in childhood or a shingles vaccine as an adult can minimize risk of developing shingles.

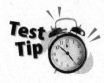

Many of the questions on the certification exam likely fall into one or both of the following categories:

1. Relates to a task that is performed frequently by paramedics.

2. Relates to a task that could harm the patient if not performed competently by the paramedic.

If it's important to know when taking care of a patient, then it's important to know before taking the certification exam.

Special Patient Populations

I. TERMS TO KNOW

A. Bariatrics—science of providing healthcare for extremely obese patients

B. Colostomy—surgical opening between colon and abdominal wall to allow passage of feces while bypassing part of colon

C. Cor pulmonale—CHF due to pulmonary hypertension

D. Fistula—surgical connection between an artery and vein for dialysis

E. Hospice—end-of-life care for the terminally ill

II. EPIDEMIOLOGY OF HOME CARE PATIENTS

A. Most are female and 65 or older.

B. Most informal caregivers (often family) spend at least four hours per day providing care, every day.

C. Medicare funding for home care is inadequate, increasing burden on EMS system.

III. COMMON EMS RESPONSE FOR HOME CARE PATIENTS

A. Equipment assistance or failure

B. Loss of caregiver

C. Transportation needed

 IV. COMMON HOME CARE MEDICAL EQUIPMENT

A. Common devices

  1. Home oxygen

  2. Tracheostomy tubes

  3. Home ventilators

  4. Apnea monitors

  5. CPAP or BiPAP machines

  6. SVN machines

  7. Surgical drains

  8. Medication infusion pumps

  9. Central IV catheters

  10. Feeding tubes

  11. Foley catheters

  12. Colostomy

  13. Peritoneal dialysis equipment

  14. Shunts and fistulas

  15. Hospital-style beds

B. General management

  1. Infection, hemorrhage, and respiratory compromise are common complications with home care devices.

  2. Stabilize immediate airway, breathing, or circulatory problems and transport.

Common Equipment Complications and EMS Management

	Common Complications	Management
Tracheostomy tube	• Mucus blockage • Dislodgement	• Suction as indicated. • Remove tube as needed. • Consider inserting ETT into stoma. • Initiate BVM as indicated.
Home ventilator	• Ventilator malfunction • Loss of electricity	• Switch to BVM.
Vascular access devices (Hickman, Broviac, Groshong)	• Infection • Accidental removal	• Control bleeding. • Transport.
Dialysis shunt	• Infection • Hemorrhage	• Do *not* apply BP cuff or start IV on same extremity. • Transport.
Urinary catheter	• Infection • Failure to drain	• Transport.

V. SPECIAL CONSIDERATIONS

A. Attempt to determine patient's normal baseline mental status.

B. Home caregivers are often more familiar with medical equipment in the home than EMS providers.

C. Be alert for signs of abuse or neglect.

D. Home care patients can have increased risk of latex sensitivity or allergy. Have latex-free equipment options readily available.

VI. SPECIFIC CONDITIONS

A. Cystic fibrosis (CF)

1. Causes chronic and copious overproduction of mucus, airway inflammation, and infections.

2. Most patients die before age 40.

3. Home management often involves manual or mechanical chest percussion.

4. Dyspnea, hemoptysis, pneumothorax, cor pulmonale are common complications.

B. Bronchopulmonary dysplasia (BPD)

1. Usually affects low birth-weight infants.

2. Often patients require continuous mechanical ventilator support.

3. Has increased risk of respiratory infections.

4. Pulmonary edema develops easily with excessive fluid administration.

C. Muscular dystrophy

1. Causes muscle degeneration and atrophy.

2. Patients often have difficulty ambulating.

3. Most EMS calls relate to respiratory problems or fall injuries.

D. Guillain-Barré syndrome

1. Autoimmune disorder causing muscle weakness leading to paralysis.

2. Paralysis starts in distal extremities and moves to core, risking respiratory paralysis.

3. Affects motor function more than sensory function.

4. Recoverable with adequate ventilatory support.

E. Myasthenia gravis

1. Causes weakness and fatigue of voluntary muscles (rare disorder).

2. Respiratory compromise possible, often preceded by difficulty swallowing or dyspnea.

F. Homelessness and poverty

1. Causes increased risk of poor health, mental health problems.

2. Advocate for patient.

3. Provide information about available community resources.

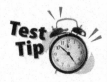

Memorizing all those flashcards you are (hopefully) making is a lot of work, but it's worth it! Treat each flashcard like it's going to earn you one more correct answers on the certification exam. Try to memorize 5–10 new flashcards each day. Set aside time every day to review the flashcards you've already memorized.

PART VII

EMS OPERATIONS

Ground and Air Ambulance Operations

I. TERMS TO KNOW

A. Cleaning — removing visible contaminants from a surface

B. Defensive driving — utilization of safe practices for vehicle operations in spite of surrounding conditions and the actions of others

C. Disinfection — use of a chemical to kill pathogens (there are low, medium, and high levels of disinfection)

D. Due regard — emergency vehicle operators are expected to drive safely at all times and may be held to a higher standard than other drivers

E. Sterilization — removal of all microbial contamination

F. System status management — uses data to anticipate demand for emergency services and adjusts staffing levels and staging locations accordingly

II. GROUND AMBULANCE OPERATIONS

A. Ambulance designs

  1. Type I: truck cab-chassis with modular ambulance body

  2. Type II: standard van with integral cab-body ambulance

  3. Type III: specialty van with integral cab-body ambulance

  4. Heavy-duty emergency vehicle

B. Ambulance minimum standards

1. Separate compartment for driver and patient/attendant

2. Room for at least two patients and attendants

3. Stocked with all required equipment and supplies (per state standards)

4. Radio communication with dispatchers

5. Ability to contact medical direction

6. Meets all federal, state, local safety standards

7. Meets state standards for state certified ambulance

8. Typically displays "star of life" emblem

C. Phases of an ambulance call

1. Preparation

   i.   Conduct ambulance inspection at start of shift.

2. Dispatch

   i.   Obtain essential information (location, MOI/NOI, etc.).

   ii. Notify dispatch you are en-route.

3. Travel to scene

   i.   Perform a safe response with due regard and defensive driving habits.

   ii. Intersections are dangerous!

4. Patient contact

   i.   Notify dispatch you are on-scene.

   ii. Position ambulance for safe patient loading.

5. Transfer to ambulance

   i.   Safely transfer and load patient in ambulance (*not* exposed to oncoming traffic).

6. Transport to receiving facility

   i.   Notify dispatch you are en-route.

   ii. Provide a safe transport to appropriate receiving facility.

        iii. Intersections are dangerous!

        iv. Ensure patient(s) and attendant(s) are properly secured.

  7. Transfer of care

        i. Notify dispatch you are at the hospital.

        ii. Provide verbal and written transfer of care report.

  8. Return to service

        i. Decontaminate ambulance and restock as indicated.

> **Note:** Review disinfection levels, Chapter 14

        ii. Notify dispatch you are back in service.

D. Due regard

  1. Emergency vehicle operators can, typically, disregard most traffic laws when responding in emergency mode.

  2. Emergency vehicle operators are required to exercise due regard at all times.

  3. *Never:*

        i. speed through a school zone.

        ii. pass a school bus with stop sign extended.

        iii. cross railroad tracks with gates down.

E. Escorts and multiple-vehicle responses

  1. Police escorts are *not* recommended unless needed for scene safety or you are lost.

  2. Exercise extreme caution with multiple-vehicle responses, especially at intersections. Likelihood of encountering another emergency vehicle increases as responding vehicles approach the scene.

F. Defensive driving tactics

  1. Do *not* sacrifice safety for speed.

  2. Know your route.

3. All occupants should be properly restrained during ambulance operations.

4. All equipment should be secured (no potential projectiles).

5. Use daytime running lights.

6. Use both lights and siren when driving in emergency mode.

7. Always know what is next to you while driving.

8. Maintain safe following distance.

9. Avoid backing up whenever possible, and always use a spotter.

10. Scan the road continuously.

11. Don't tunnel vision on vehicle directly in front of you.

12. Anticipate unexpected actions from other drivers.

13. Minimize distractions while driving.

14. Assume other drivers do not see or hear you.

15. Know your blind spots.

16. Pass on the left whenever possible.

17. Stop at all red lights, clear all intersections.

18. Account for ambulance's higher center of gravity and increased braking distance.

19. Exercise extreme caution in intersections, at night, and during inclement weather.

20. Do not develop lights and sirens "lead foot."

21. Recognize fatigue as one of the biggest threats to safe vehicle operation.

III. AIR AMBULANCE OPERATIONS

A. Types of air ambulances

1. Rotor-wing (helicopters)

   i. Used for scene calls and local interfacility transports.

2. Fixed-wing (plane/jet)

   i. Typically used for interfacility transports over 100 miles.

B. Landing zones (LZ) for rotor-wing aircraft

1. Keep LZ clear on approach and during takeoff. Aircraft may return to LZ unexpectedly and abruptly due to mechanical problems.

2. LZ should be at least 75' × 75' (day) and 100' × 100' (night) on firm, level ground and clear of overhead obstructions.

3. Ensure LZ is clear of loose debris that could be caught in rotor wash.

4. Do not light LZ with caution tape, flares, unweighted lights, or blinding strobes.

5. Establish and maintain radio contact with aircraft during approach, landing, and takeoff.

C. Working around EMS helicopters

1. Never approach aircraft without the pilot's permission.

2. Never approach aircraft from the rear.

3. Secure all loose items on patient, stretcher, and EMS personnel (hats, blankets, etc.)

4. Follow local protocols regarding appropriate use of EMS helicopters and rotor-wing safety.

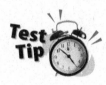

Test Tip

You are likely to see fewer EMS Operations questions on the exam than the other categories; however, you still need to prepare for this topic. Make sure you are familiar with NIMS (National Incident Management System), triage standards, and safety considerations for all types of EMS operations.

Incident Management

TERMS TO KNOW

A. NIMS—National Incident Management System

B. Closed incident—aka contained incident. Incident where injuries have already occurred prior to arrival of rescue personnel

C. Primary triage—takes place early during incident, when patients are first encountered

D. Safety officer (SO)—monitors all on-scene activities to identify and prevent harmful conditions

E. Secondary triage—ongoing triage completed throughout incident

F. Singular command—single individual has command of incident. Usually used for single-jurisdiction incidents.

G. Span of control—number of people or tasks that one individual can manage

H. Staging—positioning of resources, such as ambulances, to allow coordinated access to scene and egress from scene with patients

I. START triage—simple triage and rapid treatment

J. Triage—sorting patients based on severity of injury

K. Unified command—multiple personnel from different jurisdictions share command

II. NATIONAL INCIDENT MANAGEMENT SYSTEM (NIMS)

A. Purpose and origin

1. Standards set by Department of Homeland Security (DHS)

2. Comprehensive national approach to incident management

3. Applicable at all jurisdictional levels and across functional disciplines

4. Useful on full spectrum of incidents, regardless of size, location or complexity ·

5. Designed to be adaptable and flexible

B. NIMS priorities

1. Life safety

2. Incident stabilization

3. Property conservation

C. Command staff

1. Incident command

i. Incident commander is responsible for overall management of the incident.

ii. Command may be singular or unified.

iii. Ideal span of control should not exceed five people or tasks (never more than seven).

iv. Four sections under Command utilized as needed to maintain span of control

➤ Finance and administration

➤ Logistics

> Operations

> Planning

2. Safety officer—has authority to stop any action deemed an immediate life threat.

3. Liaison officer—Coordinates incident operations involving outside agencies.

4. Information officer—Collects incident data and communicates with media.

D. Organization of EMS operations

1. Incident command

   i. Operations

      > EMS branch

      > Triage

      > Treatment

      > Transportation

E. Triage

1. START and JumpSTART triage

   i. START Triage (adults)—see START Triage algorithm (on the next page).

   ii. JumpSTART (peds)—see Chapter 25.

2. Triage tags

   i.   Alerts other rescuers which patients have been previously triaged.

   ii. Identifies patient's triage category.

   iii. Allows tracking of patients from primary triage through transport.

   iv. Should be able to triage a patient in under 30 seconds.

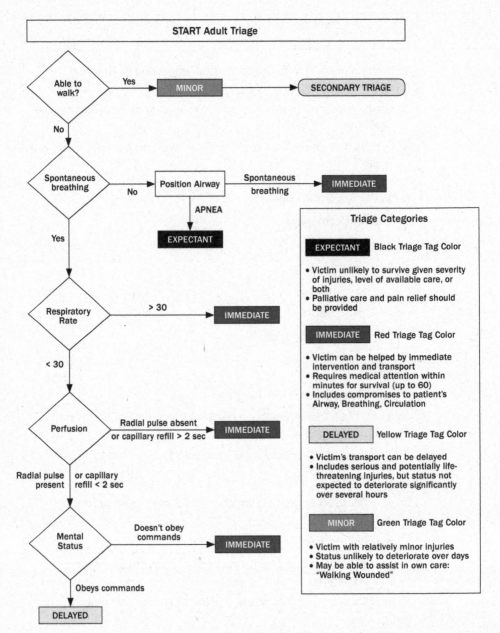

Source: U.S. National Library of Medicine

III. DISASTER MENTAL HEALTH SERVICES

A. Replaces Critical Incident Stress Management (CISM).

B. Focuses on meeting basic human needs

1. Listening, compassion

2. Ensuring basic physical needs met

3. No forced talking or sharing

4. Encouraging social support

5. Protecting from additional harm

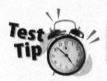

Safety first! You are likely to see several safety-related questions on the certification exam. An answer choice related to your safety is usually the correct response.

Rescue Ops, Hazmat, Terrorism

I. TERMS TO KNOW

A. Biotoxin—poisonous substance produced by living organism, such as ricin and botulinum toxin (botox)

B. CBRNE—chemical, biological, radiological, nuclear, explosives

C. Complex access—requires use of special tools and training to access/extricate patient

D. Cribbing—using timber to temporarily support weight of an object during rescue operations

E. Dirty bomb—a nuclear weapon improvised from radioactive nuclear waste material and conventional explosives

F. Emergency move—used when dangers require immediate movement of the patient

G. Entrapment—being trapped in an enclosed space

H. Extrication—removal of a patient from entrapment

I. Incapacitating agents—used for riot control or personal protection, such as mace and pepper spray

J. Incendiary agents—explosives with less power but greater heat and burn potential, such as Napalm

K. Pulmonary agents—chemical agents that damage the lungs, such as phosgene, chlorine, and hydrogen sulfide

L. Recirculating currents—movement of currents over a uniform obstruction, aka "drowning machine"

M. Safety data sheets (SDS)—contain detailed information about all hazardous substances on site (formerly called material safety data sheets (MSDS))

N. Shoring—provides temporary support of damaged or collapsed structure in order to conduct search and rescue operations

O. Simple access—gaining access to the patient without tools or breaking glass

P. Urgent move—used when patient has potential life threats and must be moved quickly

Q. Vesicant—blistering chemical agent, such as mustard gas, lewisite, and phosgene oxime

II. EMS ROLE DURING SPECIAL OPERATIONS

A. Many incidents require personnel with specialized training. Do not attempt operations for which you have not been trained.

B. EMS providers' primary role is personal safety and patient care once it is safe to do so.

C. Always wear PPE appropriate for the situation.

D. Special operations may include

1. Vehicle extrication.

2. Search and rescue/technical rescue.

3. Water rescue.

4. Structure fire.

5. Law enforcement operations.

6. Hazmat incidents.

7. Natural disasters.

8. MCIs.

III. EXTRICATION OPERATIONS

A. Scene safety

1. Leather gloves should be worn over (not instead of) regular PPE gloves when working around glass, sharp objects, rope, etc.

2. Federal law requires use of an approved, highly reflective, traffic safety vest when working on roadways, near traffic, or at an accident scene.

B. Vehicle safety systems

1. Shock-absorbing bumpers

   i. Assume all modern vehicles are equipped with shock-absorbing bumpers, front and rear.

   ii. Compressed bumpers can spontaneously release with great force.

   iii. Approach damaged vehicle from sides, not front or rear.

   iv. Do not conduct patient care in front of or behind a damaged vehicle.

2. Safety restraint systems (SRS)

   i. Assume all modern vehicles are equipped with multiple SRS airbags (up to 10 is not uncommon).

   ii. Airbags deploy at about 200 mph and could be triggered accidentally following an accident (even after battery disconnected).

   iii. Maintain safe distance (about 2') between you and undeployed airbags.

   iv. Front airbags typically deflate quickly. Side-impact airbags may deflate more slowly.

C. Phases of extrication

1. Arrival and scene size-up

    i.   Position vehicle to improve scene safety.

    ii.   Perform 360-degree walk-around if able.

    iii. Determine scene hazards, number of patients, additional resources needed.

2. Control of hazards

    i.   Traffic, fuel leaks, etc.

    ii.   Do not attempt to disconnect car battery unless trained to do so.

    iii. Electric, hybrid, and alternative fuel vehicles can present special hazards.

    ➤ All orange cables on a gasoline-electric hybrid vehicle are high voltage. However, not all high-voltage cables on a hybrid are orange.

3. Patient access

    i.   Do not attempt to gain access without proper training.

    ii.   Keep patient safe while rescuers conduct extrication ops, e.g., blanket, eye protection.

4. Patient care

    i.   Patient care can be performed during extrication ops if safe to do so.

5. Disentanglement

    i.   Simple or complex access (Do not attempt complex access without proper training and equipment.)

    ii.   Perform emergency move or urgent move as indicated.

6. Patient packaging

    i.   Complete or repeat primary assessment.

    ii.   Manage immediate life threats.

    iii. Determine transport priority.

    iv.   Complete thorough patient assessment (while en route if indicated).

7. Transport.

IV. HAZARDOUS MATERIALS

A. Hazardous materials training

1. Awareness—trains responders to recognize potential hazards. Federal law requires all rescue personnel to receive Awareness level training. (Additional info: *https://training.fema.gov*)

2. Operations—trains first responders to protect people, property, and the environment. Trained in use of specialized PPE.

3. Technician—provides significant training related to halting release or spread of hazardous materials.

4. Specialist—highest level of training. Typically provides assistance at command level.

B. Scene safety considerations

1. Hazardous materials come in many forms. Utilize all your senses to stay alert. When in doubt, get out!

2. All EMS providers should have at least Awareness level hazmat training. (*https://training.fema.gov*)

3. EMS personnel tasks on a hazmat scene include personal safety, notification of appropriate authorities, safety of the public, and patient care in a safe zone.

C. Hazmat resources

1. Emergency Response Guidebook (ERG)

2. Shipping papers

3. Safety data sheets

4. Local hazmat teams

5. CAMEO database (*https://www.epa.gov/cameo*)

6. Hazmat hotlines (CHEMTREC, CHEMTEL)

7. Poison control centers/toxicologists (1–800–222–1222 or *www.poison.org*)

D. Placards

1. Transport of hazardous materials

   i. Vehicles containing hazardous materials in certain quantities are required to display diamond-shaped identification placards.

      ➤ Placards contain a four-digit United Nations (UN) identification number.

      ➤ All UN numbers are listed in ERG.

      ➤ Report placard information when requesting additional resources—if safe to do so.

   ii. Drivers transporting hazardous materials are required to have shipping papers that identify the substance(s) and quantities being shipped.

   Note: Always be alert for hazardous materials in non-placarded vehicles (pool cleaners, exterminators, etc.).

2. Fixed storage locations

   i. Diamond placards are used for fixed storage locations with hazardous materials. Placard contains four smaller placards within it.

      ➤ Blue diamond—provides information about health hazards (numbered 0–4).

      ➤ Red diamond—provides information about fire hazard (numbered 0–4).

      ➤ Yellow diamond—provides information about reactivity hazards (numbered 0–4).

      ➤ White diamond—displays symbols indicating special hazards (radioactivity, reactive to water, etc.).

   ii. Numbering—the higher the number, the greater the hazard

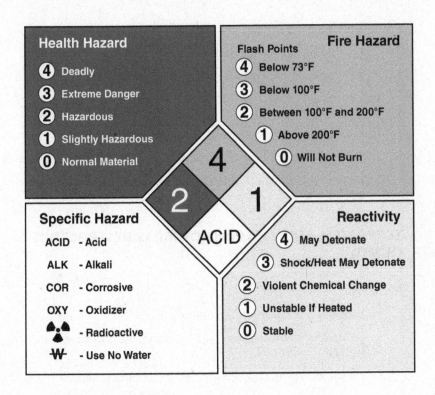

E. Hazmat zones

   1. Hot zone

      i. Contaminated area, requires appropriate PPE

        ➤ Those without proper training and PPE are *not* permitted in the hot zone. Only properly trained entry team personnel may enter the hot zone, and only for rescue or hazard mitigation.

      ii. Patient care does *not* take place in the hot zone.

   2. Warm zone

      i. Between hot and cold zones

      ii. Appropriate PPE required

      iii. Only life-threatening conditions are treated in warm zone.

      iv. Everyone in warm zone must be decontaminated in warm zone before entering cold zone.

3. Cold zone

    i.   Most treatment performed in cold zone.

    ii. Typically, EMS providers remain in cold zone.

F. Decontamination

    1. Is essential to prevent spread of hazardous material.

    2. Includes patient's hair, body, clothes, and any medical equipment.

    3. Decon should be performed by personnel trained and equipped to do so.

 V. TERRORISM AND WEAPONS OF MASS DESTRUCTION (WMD)

A. Safety considerations

    1. Your safety is *always* the first priority.

    2. Be alert for chemical, biological, radiological, nuclear, explosive (CBRNE) hazards.

    3. Follow local protocols and incident command system (ICS).

B. Chemical agents

    1. Nerve agents

        i.   Are a significant threat due to relative ease of acquisition and deployment.

        ii. Cause excessive (potentially fatal) overstimulation of the sympathetic nervous system.

        iii. Are readily available organophosphates (pesticides) that can be used as nerve agents.

        iv. Common organophosphate nerve agents include Sarin, Soman, Tabun, VX.

        v. Signs and symptoms (SLUDGEM) and management of nerve agent exposure: see Chapter 13

2. Vesicants (blistering agent)

   i. Cause pain, burns, and blisters to skin, eyes, and respiratory tract.

   ii. Onset can be immediate, or delayed several hours.

   iii. Affected areas should be irrigated with copious amounts of water ASAP.

3. Cyanide (blood agent)

   i. Signs, symptoms, and management: see Chapter 13

4. Pulmonary (choking) agents

   i. Cause dyspnea, cough, wheezing, sore throat.

   ii. Manage ABCs, administer oxygen, ventilate as indicated, consider bronchodilator meds.

C. Biological agents

   1. Are used to cause disease.

   2. Examples—anthrax, pneumonic plague, tularemia, smallpox

   3. Can cause fever, weakness, flu-like symptoms, respiratory distress.

   4. Require supportive care.

D. Radiological/nuclear weapons

   1. See Chapter 19

E. Explosives

   1. Most commonly used WMD

   2. Expect significant blunt and penetrating trauma, burns, and crush injuries.

      i. Primary blast injuries—injuries caused directly by the blast wave (pressure wave)

      ii. Secondary blast injuries—injuries caused by shrapnel and flying debris

      iii. Tertiary blast injuries—injuries caused by striking the ground or other objects

F. Incapacitating agents

1. Agents intentionally designed to incapacitate without permanent injury.

2. Often used by law enforcement or for personal protection; however, could also be used by terrorists.

3. Signs and symptoms

   i.   Eye irritation, lacrimation (excessive tearing)

   ii. Rhinorrhea (runny nose)

   iii. Airway irritation, dyspnea

4. Management

   i.   Ensure scene safety, appropriate PPE.

   ii. Remove from source.

   iii. Administer oxygen as indicated.

   iv. Irrigation as indicated.

   ➤ Irrigate the eyes and skin as indicated for 10–20 minutes.

   ➤ Remove contact lenses.

   ➤ Use water or normal saline solution.

   ➤ Do not pour over forehead (can contaminate eyes).

   ➤ Do not force eyes open.

   ➤ Once eyes treated, have patient close eyes and irrigate entire head to prevent secondary contamination of eyes.

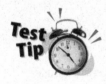

Test Tip

If you would like to learn more about the EMS aspects of terrorism response and WMD, visit https://training.fema.gov/ *and complete the free online IS-100.C: Introduction to the Incident Command System course. Here are two additional recommended courses through* www.teex.org:

- **AWR111:** *Basic Emergency Medical Services (EMS) Concepts for Chemical, Biological, Radiological, Nuclear, and Explosive (CBRNE) Events*

- **AWR160:** *WMD/Terrorism Awareness for Emergency Responders*

The Paramedic Psychomotor Exam

Once you've completed and passed your cognitive exam, you'll need to take and pass the paramedic psychomotor exam.

I. SKILLS TESTED ON THE NREMT PARAMEDIC PSYCHOMOTOR EXAM

Paramedic candidates are tested on six skills during the psychomotor exam:

- ➤ Patient Assessment: Trauma
- ➤ Dynamic Cardiology
- ➤ Static Cardiology
- ➤ Oral Station Case A
- ➤ Oral Station Case B
- ➤ Integrated Out-of-Hospital Scenario

II. TOP 10 TIPS TO PREPARE FOR THE PARAMEDIC PSYCHOMOTOR EXAM

1. Determine the specifics about the psychomotor examination process in your state.

2. Obtain all available skill sheets that will be used for your psychomotor exam and know them. Know them cold!

3. Make sure your ECG (electrocardiogram) and ACLS (advanced cardiac life support) skills are sharp. Be able to quickly verbalize treatment for both stable and unstable patients with cardiac dysrhythmias (examples: VF/PVT, narrow and wide-complex tachycardias, bradycardias, asystole, PEA)

4. Practice to proficiency! There is no substitute for this. Practicing a couple of times is like doing a couple of sit-ups—NOT MUCH HELP! Practice and repeat. Practice and repeat. This is the single best way to reduce the stress of high-stakes testing. Why don't you get nervous while driving any longer? PRACTICE!

5. If there are opportunities in your area to immerse yourself in a practice environment the week or so leading up to your practical exam—do it!

6. Listen carefully to the instructions provided in each station. These instructions contain valuable information and include the time limit for the station.

7. If given the opportunity to review or organize your equipment before the station begins, do it.

8. Don't overlook the BLS (basic life support) skills that may be included in your practical exam. It's not unusual for paramedic candidates to have trouble with a BLS skill rather than an ALS (advanced life support) skill.

9. Articulate! Do what you say, and say what you do. Your brain, hands, and voice should all be working at the same time.

10. Stay calm. Trust your abilities. Focus only on the one station in front of you. Forget about the previous station, or the next station.

For additional information about the NREMT psychomotor exam, visit the NREMT website.